Tongue-Tie... Roundtable

Edited by
Kathleen Kendall-Tackett, PhD, IBCLC, RLC, FAPA
Marsha Walker, RN, IBCLC, RLC
Catherine Watson Genna, BS, IBCLC, RLC

All royalties go to the
U.S. Lactation Consultant Association.

Praeclarus Press, LLC
©2018. United States Lactation Consultant Association

Praeclarus Press, LLC
2504 Sweetgum Lane
Amarillo, Texas 79124 USA
806-367-9950
www.PraeclarusPress.com

DISCLAIMER

The information contained in this publication is advisory only and is not intended to replace sound clinical judgment or individualized patient care. The author disclaims all warranties, whether expressed or implied, including any warranty as the quality, accuracy, safety, or suitability of this information for any particular purpose.

ISBN: 978-1-946665-14-0

Cover Design: Ken Tackett
Acquisition & Development: Kathleen Kendall-Tackett
Copy Editing: Kathleen Kendall-Tackett & Chris Tackett
Layout & Design: Nelly Murariu

Contents

Introduction

The Tongue-tie controversy. How shall we then treat?

For many years, I've watched as experts in tongue-tie fought to get health care providers to recognize its existence. I still remember Cathy Watson Genna and Donna Geddes showing ultrasound videos of before and after a tongue-tie release. They made believers out of everyone in the room. Finally, at least some health care providers were recognizing tongue-tie, and were willing to do something about it.

More recently, however, I've seen the controversy surrounding tongue-tie grow, particularly on social media. The conversation has become so polarized that dissenting voices are shouted down, and people have even lost their jobs when they dared to differ from the prevailing orthodoxy.

How did we get here?
And what should our next steps be?

Caught in the middle of this mess are mothers, babies, and the IBCLCs who are trying to help them. That is why we have this roundtable on tongue-tie. We identified practitioners who are experts. We asked them to participate, and they graciously agreed.

What Should Our Goals Be
Regarding Tongue-Tie?

When talking about an important clinical issue, we need to keep our goals in mind. Regarding tongue-tie, there are three important goals we have identified.

1. **Helping mothers achieve pain-free breastfeeding.** When mothers say that they are in pain, we need to hear them. So many mothers tell practitioners that they are in pain, and the practitioners either ignore them, or say, "it should get better eventually." Those responses are not acceptable. *Pain means something is wrong*, and tongue-tie might be the cause. It isn't always, but it is something we should consider.

   Some mothers think pain means *they* are doing something wrong. We also need to communicate that this is not their fault. We should let mothers know that we will work with them to figure out what is causing their pain so that breastfeeding will stop hurting. I believe that practitioners ignoring mothers' pain has led to much of what is happening on social media. We need to listen to what they are trying to say.

2. **Helping babies get enough to eat.** Mothers also reported that their babies were on the breast "all the time," never seemed satisfied, and had faltering weight gains. Again, these struggles were minimized, and then mothers were told to supplement. In some cases, supplementing may have been necessary in the short term, as the babies may have been struggling and no one picked it up until there was a crisis. However, the mothers' stories reveal that babies' struggles to transfer enough milk were also ignored or minimized. A baby on "all the time" should also be evaluated. A tongue-tie is one possible reason, and it is a direct threat to the mother's milk production.

3. **Protecting breastfeeding.** The mothers' stories we share are heart-breaking. It's amazing that these mothers persisted and continued breastfeeding. In some cases,

the difficulties they encountered led to insufficient milk, and they never regained a full supply. Keep in mind that the stories we share are only from the mothers who continued. How many more did we lose along the way? If we want mothers to exclusively breastfeed for 6 months, we need to hear what they are trying to tell us. Tongue-tie might be one reason why they are struggling, so it's important for us to consider.

Important Questions

In addition to our goals, IBCLCs need answers to several practical questions.

1. If we suspect a tongue-tie, how should we assess the baby?

2. What are the best and most-effective ways to treat tongue-tie? Where do we send mothers for treatment? How can we address tongue-tie in the least intrusive way?

3. What should be done for after care?

4. Are there alternatives to surgery?

Tongue-tie also raises some important Scope of Practice issues for IBCLCs. We are often the only practitioners to recognize a tongue-tie, and obviously, can't ignore it. What should be our role?

The Expert Panel and Roundtable

With these questions in mind, we assembled our panel of experts. We first identified people we knew who had international reputations as experts on tongue-tie. Our panelists suggested other experts to contact. We made sure that the panel represented a wide range of disciplines (pediatrics, family medicine, dentistry, craniosacral therapy, speech and language pathology, and research). Most of our experts were also IBCLCs, and were from the U.S., Brazil, Australia, and Spain.

Roundtable Format

About 10 years ago, I attended a session at American Psychological Association on the topic of cancer and posttraumatic stress disorder (PTSD). One speaker laid out all his reasons why he thought cancer caused PTSD. The next speaker laid out all his reasons why he thought it didn't. They didn't argue with each other. They simply presented their views. Both made many excellent points, and I found the conversation to be quite helpful. I have used that format to address other controversial questions, such as whether prospective or retrospective findings were most accurate in child maltreatment research. Those articles get cited a lot.

We have adopted a similar format here. We assembled a list of questions and asked our panelists to answer them. These are practitioners whose opinions we trust, and we know that they have the best interests of mothers and babies in mind. You will see that they don't always agree with each other in how to best address the issues they encounter. Our goal is not consensus, but to show where we are now. Our experts disagreed the most on posterior tongue-tie and post-revision care. Even with disagreement, however, the conversation was civil and professional—exactly where we need it to be for us to move forward. It's helpful to see the views side by side.

We have also asked Liz Brooks to discuss Scope of Practice for IBCLCs regarding tongue-tie, including the most current guidelines. Mothers' stories are also part of this discussion, so we have included those as well. Finally, we have included some clinical pictures, links to videos, and two assessment tools.

We think this issue is a step towards reaching a consensus on this controversial issue. I think you will be impressed with the depth of our panelists' knowledge, and their obvious compassion for mothers and babies.

We hope that this discussion is helpful in your practice. That has always been our chief goal for the journal. Thank you for helping mothers meet these challenges and attain their breastfeeding goals.

Kathleen Kendall-Tackett, PhD, IBCLC, RLC, FAPA
Editor-in-Chief

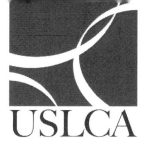

USLCA

Incidence and Prevalence of Tongue-Tie

Keywords: tongue-tie, incidence, prevalence

What is the prevalence of tongue-tie (the proportion of total cases in a population)? Is the incidence (occurrence of new cases) increasing or are clinicians simply identifying it more often? The most reliable way to estimate incidence and prevalence is through population-based epidemiologic studies. So far, these are limited. However, there has been some research that allows us to approximate rates. Our expert panel offers their judgment on two questions. What is the approximate percentage of babies with tongue-tie? And is incidence increasing?

The Percentage of Infants with Tongue-Tie

Alison Hazelbaker

The exact prevalence of tongue-tie is unknown. According to the current body of evidence, prevalence rates range from 0.1% to 10%, clustering around 3.5-5%, depending on the criteria used to evaluate the lingual frenum in a particular study. The highest and lowest numbers occur when visual criteria dominate the assessment process, for example, lowest percentage when using thick visible frenum on lift (Sedano, 1975) and highest percentage when using the Hogan-Westcott-Griffiths classification schema (2005). This variability suggests that the assessment processes in these two studies was nonspecific in the former (false negatives), and nonsensitive in the latter (false positives).

Prevalence testing was only undertaken relatively recently when David Todd, an Australian neonatologist, mounted a 3-year study that screened every baby born in his facility using a standardized assessment tool.

In a sample size of 9,478 babies, he found that an average of 4.83% of babies per year were tongue-tied requiring surgery. Another 5% had signs but were able to normalize function with management alone. According to the definition of true tongue-tie, this amounts to a prevalence statistic of about 5%. Further, 70% of the truly tongue-tied babies had a ventral tongue frenum attachment in front of the body-blade juncture

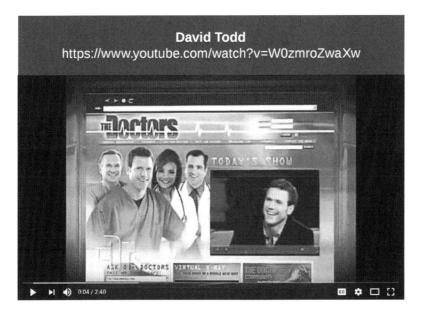

David Todd
https://www.youtube.com/watch?v=W0zmroZwaXw

(anterior tie), and only 30% had a ventral tongue attachment behind the body-blade juncture (posterior tie; Todd, 2014; Todd & Hogan, 2015).

Carmela Baeza

It varies from <1 percent to 10 percent, depending on the study population and criteria used to define it. To determine the incidence of any condition, it is requisite that it is previously defined, that there is a consensus so that the condition can be identified and reported by every healthcare professional. This is not the case with ankyloglossia. Although there is a morphological definition (a congenital anomaly in which a short, lingual frenulum restricts tongue movement), there is no consensus as to its different types and its clinical impact, and therefore, it is not homogeneously reported. It is therefore difficult to be sure whether its incidence is increasing or rather the awareness of its impact in the breastfeeding dyad is (Gonzalez Jimenez et al., 2014; Hall & Renfrew, 2005; Mueller & Callahan, 2007; Segal, Stephenson, Dawes, & Feldman., 2007).

Catherine Watson Genna

I only see infants having breastfeeding difficulties, so it's unsurprising that I see a higher incidence of tongue-tie than that reported in the literature, which ranges from 3.5% to 13%. We would need good studies using the same well-standardized assessment on similar populations a decade or two apart to determine if the incidence is increasing. This would be particularly difficult because we don't know what we don't know yet.

James Murphy

While at a teaching hospital with 325 births per month, I saw 15% of the newborns each month for release of tongue-ties and still had lots of complaints that other newborns could not get an appointment with me to release a tongue-tie. I estimate the true incidence of tongue-movement restriction that would benefit by surgical release to be roughly 20-25%. This would include all such movement restrictions regardless of what "type" it is felt to be. I was fairly selective about which restrictions I would release when I started doing this in 2003. Some of the infants I elected not to release came back later with more significant clinical symptoms which resolved when I then agreed to release the restriction. Thus, I gradually included more and more of those who I previously felt were too "mild" to release. I now know that if there is at least a small, midline mouth floor "speed bump" detected by little finger sweep from side to side and the usual clinical symptoms of tongue-tie are present, this constitutes a restriction that should be released.

The concept of mild, moderate, and severe tongue-ties based on visual appearance is false. The condition must be assessed on the severity of interference with normal breastfeeding. Some questions include: is mom's milk production increasing to the level needed to meet the caloric needs of the infant(s)? Is a nursing session less than 40 min and satisfies the infant(s) for at least 2-3 hours? Is the latch comfortable for mom and not damaging to mom's breast tissues? Is the infant(s) able to transfer milk efficiently and gaining weight as expected? As we consider all of these factors, and not just the appearance of the tongue and mouth floor, we likely are including more infants in the category of clinically significant tongue-tie, and thus the "incidence" of tongue-tie is likely enlarging in parallel with our understanding of what constitutes a tongue-tie.

Martin Kaplan

Currently, the most consistent ranges that I encounter are from 1.7%-12% of the examined general population, but can be as high as 25% in infants with breastfeeding problems. This answer is based on the various publications, texts and educational workshops that I have attended. However, I do believe there have not been consistent standardized reproducible evaluator guidelines for these numbers, so they are highly variable.

Historically, I was one of the few pediatric dentists in the 1970s to learn the basic bladed frenotomy procedure, while a clinical chief resident during my pediatric dental training at a major hospital in NYC. The guidelines for treatment were very subjective. Simply put, if you could not speak well, or if there was a big gap between the teeth after orthodontic treatment, then a surgical revision was necessary. At no time were babies and toddlers ever considered for evaluation. If there was any major tongue surgery for a release, this was under the pervue of either ENT (ear, nose, and throat) or oral surgery to perform an involved Z-plasty. So, the standards that I was trained by are based on older guidelines, and are not based on current standards for identifying frenum restrictions that we are discussing in this forum.

Pamela Douglas

From the 1950s, classic (or anterior) tongue-tie (CTT) was often overlooked as a cause of breastfeeding problems. In a literature review in 2005, Hall and Renfrew acknowledged that the true prevalence of ankyloglossia remained unknown, though they estimated 3-4% of newborns.

After 2005, once the diagnosis of posterior tongue-tie (PTT) had been introduced (Coryllos et al., 2004), attempts to quantify incidence have remained of very poor quality, but estimates currently rest at between 4-10% (National Health and Medical Research Council, 2012).

The problem is that there is a lack of definitional clarity concerning the diagnosis of PTT, and CTT is now often conflated with PTT, as simply "tongue-tie" (TT). Between 2004 and 2013, the incidence of TT diagnosis in Canada increased by 70%; the rate of frenotomy increased by 90%. In Australia, emerging epidemiological data shows an exponential rise in the incidence of Medicare-funded frenotomies since 2008, and this data does not even consider laser surgery by dentists, who perhaps perform a majority of frenotomies (Kapoor, 2017; Wattis et al., 2017).

Fortunately, CTTs are now much less likely to be overlooked! But this kind of pattern is recognized by epidemiologists as typical of over-treatment.

The absence of baseline data telling us about the normal spectrum of newborn oral connective tissue variation underscores how matters related to clinical breastfeeding support are still not a health system or research priority. In fact, I'd argue that this lack of investment is the *actual* story that underlies the oral ties controversy.

Roberta Martinelli and Irene Marchesan

There are several definitions of tongue-tie, as well several assessment tools reported in the literature. That fact makes the calculation of incidence rates more difficult as each professional or health center has different assessing criteria. For knowing the real incidence of tongue-tie, there should be standardization of tongue-tie definitions and standardization of validated protocols. In Brazil, Lingual Frenulum Protocols have been validated in order to provide standardized assessment criteria and consequently provide more accurate incidence data.

Is Incidence of Tongue-Tie Increasing?

Martin Kaplan

I do not have evidence to quote that the incidence is either higher or lower. I think we have just not given the proper attention in an intake health questionnaire or physical examination, and therefore we have not diagnosed accurately. If I was not educated in the evaluation of these frenum-related issues, I would have continued to assume the numbers of treatment necessary cases over the past 10+ years would be the same low numbers that I saw over my career prior to that.

I now see hundreds of babies for necessary treatment for restrictive frenum. So, the incidence to me suddenly went from zero babies to hundreds a year. Was this a sudden developmental crisis or infectious disease-like epidemic, or was this there all along and I just was not aware of its existence?

I do find that I have been treating an almost unending stream of patients, from newborns to mature adults, who all have tongue-tie issues that were unrecognized for the entirely of their life. Based on the number of the referrals to my practice, you would think that over 90% of the referred population has a tongue-tie.

We absolutely must re-examine the way we presently identify tongue and also lip frenum, and how it impacts the apparent increase in numbers of treated cases we are presently seeing clinically, and reading about on social media. There, essentially, never was any contact with any breastfeeding-related problems, or how to work with an IBCLC. The current IBCLC and social-media-infant referrals are coming to me because they have exhausted the simple fixes that help with breastfeeding using position adjustment for baby and nipple, nipple shields, accessory feeders, and elimination diets for the mother due to reflux symptoms, and oral and nasal infant leakage. These compensations were no longer sustainable, and thus the increased referral base.

Christina Smillie

This should be a simple question, but it is not, because definitions of tongue-tie vary so much. Based on my clinical experience over the past 21 years in an exclusively breastfeeding-medicine tertiary practice, I do NOT believe the incidence is increasing. I do believe our professional sensitivity to looking for restricted functional lingual mobility has increased, but I don't have any evidence that this means there has been any true change in the epidemiology of this issue within the infant population. Since I'm in a tertiary setting, I don't have a good basic denominator upon which to judge my numerator. I have seen referrals to evaluate for posterior tongue-tie increase over the past decade, but a good chunk of these are babies who are having the same variety of breastfeeding problems I have always seen, who also happen to have the same posterior frenulum that 95% of the population has, but with no actual restricted lingual function. Not that the posterior oral tissues can't be restrictive. They certainly can, but the recent increased "diagnosis" of "posterior tongue-tie" may reflect an increased enthusiasm for the diagnosis more than an increased incidence of actual restricted function.

References

Coryllos, E., Watson Genna, C., & Salloum, A. (2004). Congenital tongue-tie and its impact on breastfeeding. Breastfeeding: Best for Mother and Baby, *American Academy of Pediatrics, Summer*, 1-6.

González Jiménez, D., Costa Romero, M., Riaño Galán, I., González Martínez, M., Rodríguez Pando, M., & Lobete Prieto, C. (2014). Prevalencia de anquiloglosia en recién nacidos en el Principado de Asturias. *An Pediatr (Barc), 81*, 115–119.

Hall, D., & Renfrew, M. (2005). Tongue tie. *Archives of Disease in Childhood, 90*, 1211-1215.

Hogan, M., Westcott, C., & Griffiths, M. (2005). Randomized, controlled trial of division of tongue-tie in infants with feeding problems. *Journal of Paediatric and Child Health, 41*, 246-250.

Kapoor, V. (2017). (Ed.) *Tied to tongue-ties. New clinical tools for early life care: the Possums conference.*

Mueller, D.T., & Callanan, V.P. (2007). Congenital malformations of the oral cavity. *Otolaryngology Clinics of North America, 40,* 141.

National Health and Medical Research Council. (2012). *Infant feeding guidelines: information for health workers.* Retrieved from: https://www.nhmrc.gov.au/ guidelines-publications/n56.

Sedano, H.O. (1975). Congenital oral anomalies in Argentinean children. *Community Dentistry and Oral Epidemiology, 3,* 61-63.

Segal, L.M., Stephenson, R., Dawes, M., & Feldman, P. (2007). Prevalence, diagnosis, and treatment of ankyloglossia: Methodologic review. *Canadian Family Physician, 53,* 1027.

Todd, D. (2014). *Tongue ties: Divide and conquer? To divide and prevent an interruption in breastfeeding.* Australian Breastfeeding Association Seminars for Health Professionals.

Todd, D., & Hogan, M.J. (2015). Tongue tie in the newborn: early diagnosis and division prevents poor breastfeeding outcomes. *Breastfeeding Review, 23*(1), 11-16.

Wattis, L., Kam, R., & Douglas, P. (2017). Three experienced lactation consultants reflect upon the oral tie phenomenon. *Breastfeeding Review, 25*(1), 9.

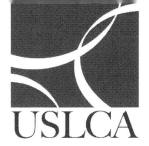

Assessment and Classification of Tongue-Tie

Keywords: tongue-tie; assessment; classification

Tongue-tie can cause many serious breastfeeding problems, and even lead to breastfeeding cessation. As the mothers' stories attest, health care providers often do not correctly identify when a baby has a tongue-tie. Assessing tongue-tie is essential, but what should clinicians look for? And which professionals should be the ones identifying tongue-tie? Assessing tongue-tie is the focus of this chapter.

How Should Tongue-Tie Be Identified?

Carmela Baeza

As I see it, there are two levels of identification. First, the morphological identification: on inspection of the baby's mouth, a short frenulum may be identified. The second level would be the clinical one: a short frenulum may or may not have an impact on the breastfeeding dyad. These two levels are frequently at odds, and I believe this is the main difficulty in the diagnosis of tongue-tie.

21

The sooner tongue-tie is identified, the better. Therefore, any health care professional who is in contact with an infant from birth should be able to identify an ankyloglossia and its clinical impact, if there is one: midwives, obstetricians, pediatricians, nurses. Lactation consultants should ideally be a second-step intervention, called on for management of unclear cases.

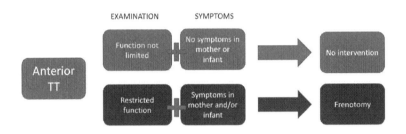

Algorithm for assessing an anterior tongue-tie. Carmela Baeza, MD, IBCLC.

Catherine Watson Genna

Every health care professional who interacts with infants and children should know how to assess for tongue attachment and function, and should do so independently to avoid confirmation bias.

James Murphy

A midline, mouth-floor palpable band of tissue that restricts normal tongue function is a tongue-tie. There may be a translucent midline "sail" connecting this fibrous band to the underside of the tongue, attaching anywhere from the tongue tip, to being just barely visible above the fibrous band.

The physical findings are a tongue tip that cannot rise or be lifted to at least 1 cm above a line connecting the mouth corners, a tongue leading edge that rises more on the sides than in the center, the tongue tip cannot extend more than ¼" past the lower lip horizontally, and may have an indentation in the midline during attempted tongue-tip extension. With the little finger pad up in the mouth of the infant, there should be a good seal, good suction with good tongue undulation. The tongue should remain on the finger during suckling as the mandible is pulled down.

The infant weight gain should be parallel to one of the normal exclusively breastfed growth curves. The duration of a full infant feeding should not exceed 40 min, and should not be needed more than every 2 to 4 hours. Mom should not experience pain during the latch session. Her nipples should remain round after the session has ended, and should not have any physical damage.

Alison Hazelbaker

Tongue-tie, by definition, is an embryological remnant of connective tissue underneath the tongue that failed to recede by apoptosis *and* that adversely impacts tongue function. Its definition is a functional one rather than based on visual criteria alone (Hazelbaker, 1993; Hazelbaker, 2010). It presents both visually, and functionally, along a continuum, and therefore has multiple visual and functional manifestations. These presentation characteristics make it difficult to design a standardized screening tool. Over-simplification of the screening process results in false negatives and positives (e.g., simply lifting the tongue to look underneath does not constitute a thorough examination nor will it accurately identify a true tongue-tie).

Assessment Tools

Differential diagnosis should proceed using a standardized, valid, reliable, sensitive and specific screening tool/process. Greenhalgh's (2014) book, *How to Read a Paper*, provides a clear explanation of each of these qualities. Only two tools qualify to date: The Assessment Tool for Lingual Frenulum Function©™ (ATLFF) (Hazelbaker, 1993, 2010), and the Lingual Frenulum Protocol for Infants, which has just undergone validity and reliability testing. (de Castro Martinelli et al., 2016). Both are included in this volume.

The ATLFF was designed to be used on all babies, regardless of feeding method. We live in a bottle-feeding culture, so the tool was designed to screen bottle-fed babies, as well as breastfed babies. The ATLFF assesses seven functional movements of the tongue, and five visual characteristics of the lingual frenum. Each of these 12 items possess sub-item characteristics to increase sensitivity and specificity. A number of 0, 1, or 2 is assigned to individual sub-items with normal characteristics assigned a 2, and significantly abnormal assigned a 0. The higher the score, the closer to normal the baby's tongue function and frenum appearance.

By looking at the final numbers in each section of the ATLFF, a diagnosis can be determined and a surgical decision can be made. A baby who scores lower than 11 on the added up function item scores, and lower than 8 on the added appearance item scores, is tongue-tied and needs surgery. A baby scoring greater than 11 to 13 on function, and 8 or 9 on appearance, either has a borderline, but functional lingual frenum, or a sucking issue from another cause. Under these circumstances, management is recommended. A baby with 14 on function (the highest possible score on the function section) is functionally normal, regardless of how the lingual frenulum visually manifests. If the tool is used correctly, no baby will score low on appearance and perfect on function. The two sections of assessment buttress one another in making an accurate tongue-tie diagnosis.

Martin Kaplan

I was never formally trained in infant tongue-tie evaluation, as there were no classes teaching how to evaluate something that was seen and treated by physicians in the delivery room. I first learned about infant frenotomy, and the related breastfeeding problems, in a pediatric laser-applications lecture at the ALD (Academy of Laser Dentistry) in 2005. I had been an active member in the academy since my training and testing in 2003. Since then, I have begun to apply my new-found knowledge with laser gum and frenum surgery to replace the bladed procedures that I was performing. This more advanced laser surgery was easily clinically transferred to infants for me, as I was already a trained pediatric dentist, and comfortable with this younger age group.

Then, my voracious appetite for more training and education for the infant tongue-tie issues led me to Alison Hazelbaker, and her book, *Tongue-tie: Morphogenesis, impact, and treatment*, which I have read and reread many times. I then was recommended, by my new IBCLC friends, to seek out Catherine Watson Genna's book, *Supporting Sucking Skills*, Marsha Walker's book, *Breastfeeding management for the clinician*, and Diana West and Lisa Marasco's text, *The Breastfeeding Mother's Guide to Making More Milk*. These are my go-to references for identifying tongue-tie related breastfeeding problems.

The most referenced studies for tongue-tie evaluation are "appearance" and "function" items based on the 1993 development of the ATLFF assessment tool. There are: Frenotomy Assessment Rule by Srinivasan etc. al., the Academy of Orofacial Myofunctional Therapy (AOMT) is currently publishing an assessment tool by Martinelli, and a few other references for tongue-tie evaluation are in the current research literature.

I found that many of these evaluation tools were not adequate for the surgical provider. Most are breastfeeding and oral-feeding-function assessments geared to lactation and feeding specialist. Since I use lasers to treat frenum, I needed an objective clinical tool to help me identify and solve the physical and functional items to decide how to treat the tissue biotypes. Since there were none, I decided to develop my own laser surgical assessment tool, which is clinically based, to help me identify tissue types for proper planning laser/tissue interaction.

As a Fellow of the Academy of Laser Dentistry (ALD), and an American Board of Laser Surgery trained diplomate, I am in constant contact with other respected laser providers of infant frenotomy, as we share our understanding with each other. I am hopeful that we can develop a universal assessment tool for providers in the very near future. We need a better assessment tool to keep our statistics for EBR (evidence-based research). The problem is also, how do you do a sham surgery?

I also ask for any reports from IBCLCs, gastroenterologists, and other physicians, and so forth, as additional supporting evidence to help identify clinically relevant frena. In my opinion, no treatment should be performed without assessing both the mother and the baby, and hopefully they have seen an IBCLC or feeding specialist along with a previous infant and breastfeeding physical exam.

Who Should Assess Tongue-Tie?

Martin Kaplan

Assessment, in my opinion, should first of all be by the attending delivery physician, midwife, doula, or an IBCLC, as they should be the first person after delivery (and ideally within the first hour) who assists the mother during the first breastfeeding. Other than the ATLFF, I do not think there are any well-researched guidelines for assessing tongue-tie that is universally and currently taught to all IBCLC or other breastfeeding-trained personnel.

As a group, physicians and dentists have very limited, if any, education on proper tongue-tie assessment. This is rapidly changing as the proper recognition of the impact on the health and well-being of the infant is finally becoming more understood. The numbers of educational classes and website opportunities are increasing in medicine and dentistry about frenum-related issues, so these two groups should be included as assessors.

Unfortunately, there is currently a large backlash from many who consider this as a "fad" diagnosis that will pass. Many mainstream health care providers believe there has been no reported benefit to the health and well-being of the baby when frena are successfully revised, even when there is an improvement, or total recovery from "aerophagia" reflux symptoms. This exists, even though there is an over usage of reflux medications, such as ranitidine, lansoprazole, and simethicone (not evidence-based; just symptoms prescribed) without clinically significant improvement. Some even believe that the current use of laser treatment is perpetuated by dental-laser companies, as a resource for more sales and income for dentists.

Roberta Martinelli and Irene Marchesan

We believe it is necessary to assess the anatomic characteristics of the tongue and lingual frenulum, and the functional aspects of the tongue, in order to have the correct diagnosis.

In Brazil, most tongue-tie assessments are performed by SLPs. However, some pediatricians, ENTs, and mainly pediatric dentists also assess lingual frenulum.

27

Pamela Douglas

All health professional groups dealing with newborns and infants need to perform oral assessments, and be capable of identifying potentially problematic lingual frenula, not just breastfeeding support professionals (BSPs). Here, I define BSPs as health professionals involved in the clinical support of breastfeeding, most commonly midwives, lactation consultants, and child health nurses. Other health professionals with special interest in clinical breastfeeding support may also be BSPs.

Alison Hazelbaker

Who should screen and diagnose? Ideally, all babies should be screened for tongue-tie within a day or two of birth, and treated if they are truly tongue-tied. Whoever examines the baby would then be the individual performing the tongue-tie screening. Since tongue-tie is not just about breastfeeding, but is a developmental issue, multiple practitioners now need to be qualified to screen since routine screening in early infancy does not occur in this and many other countries. However, each and every one of these professionals needs adequate training to perform the screening correctly so that NO baby receives an inaccurate diagnosis and the wrong treatment, potentially doing harm.

There are many children and adults who are truly tongue-tied because we do not have a mandatory screening program in the United States. Speech language pathologists and myo-functional therapists may be in the best position to perform an accurate functional assessment in children and adults. However, unless a child or adult is already going to see one of these therapists, other practitioners who more routinely see these groups should be trained to properly assess and diagnose. Unfortunately, at present, no valid or reliable screening tool is being used by physicians or dentists to accurately identify those children and adults affected by tongue-tie. This lack is partly fueling the diagnosis dilemma. Professionals are left to their own judgment and experience, at whatever level that may be, creating ripe ground for controversy and defensive debate.

Christina Smillie

I think we need to stop paying so much attention to what we see under the tongue, and pay more attention to lingual mobility and function, and in particular, the range of motion necessary for easy breastfeeding, With the mouth wide open, as the baby's jaw drops, the tongue needs to be able to get over the gingiva and lift upwards, without the either the back of the tongue, or the front being abnormally forced downwards in a way that inhibits the normal action of the tongue to move the milk.

Most of us have a stretchy posterior frenulum that does not inhibit such movement—we can eat ice cream cones and French kiss. The issue for a baby is not whether we IBCLCs can see a frenulum under the tongue, or feel it with our fingers as we pass under the tongue, but whether this posterior frenulum restricts full tongue movement for moving a bolus of milk. As for which professional groups should do this, NONE of us has been professionally trained to do this, although many of us are self-taught.

Lactation consultants, as a whole, have been trained to evaluate breastfeeding issues, but have not been trained in the ins and outs of diagnosis and differential diagnosis, and by IBLCE scope of practice rules are not technically supposed to be diagnosing anyway (but, see below.) Even without scope of practice issues, this is politically fraught. Leaving rules and regulations and politics aside, I think it is less about which profession should be doing this, and rather more about who has been trained, or self-trained, in oral anatomy and physiology, and breastfeeding and lactation issues. For anterior tongue-ties, this identification is pretty simple. But for posteriors, we want professionals who have the knowledge, and courage to make a decision when need be, while maintaining the caution to avoid jumping in where angels fear to tread.

Classifications of Tongue-Tie

Alison Hazelbaker

Through the ages, there have been many ways to classify tongue-tie. When I was performing my original research and then writing my book, I read about many different classification schemas for tongue-tie (Flinck et al., 1994; Garcia Pola et al., 2002; Kotlow, 1999; Todd-Hogan et al., 2015; Hansson; Naimer et al, 2003; and Coryllos-Watson Genna, 2016). Generally speaking, tongue-tie classification schemas use appearance criteria, rather than functional criteria, to categorize the phenomenon. These communication tools, therefore, lack the sensitivity and specificity to garner accurate diagnosis of the *functional* problem we call tongue-tie. (Greenhalgh, 2014).

Identifying a tongue-tie as either anterior or posterior is a classification schema, and today is the most commonly used classification system, surprisingly, across professions. Generally, professionals have a tendency to use classification tools authored by a member of their own profession.

My preference is to simply identify those babies with tongue-tie as being tongue-tied rather than getting hung up on what class into which they may fall. To me, it is immaterial whether the ventral tongue attachment is closer to the tip or to the base. A truly tongue-tied baby needs intervention: good feeding management and properly done surgery.

Catherine Watson Genna

Most classifications are based on appearance, which needs to be correlated with function to be meaningful. The Coryllos classification is most frequently used, it was developed to show that restrictive frenula do not necessarily extend to the tongue tip, but does not imply that any particular frenulum appearance is definitely abnormal. Dr. Coryllos always said that the tongue function had to be impaired (the tongue attachment caused a symptomatic tongue-tie), which she estimated to be about 50% of children whose tongue attachment looked too anterior or short.

James Murphy

A tongue-tie is a thick fibrous midline mouth floor band with or without a thin sail above it. The first is referred to as a posterior, or submucosal tie. The latter is an anterior tie. Using Types 1, 2, 3, & 4 describe only one aspect of the whole picture.

Martin Kaplan

Tongue-tie classifications range from anterior, posterior and the controversial "submucosal." They are also classified according to the classification of 1, 2, 3, & 4, Kotlow also has a dental tongue-tie evaluator that is useful for assessment of the appearance items to measure the ranges length of the restriction, and its impact on mobility and function.

Christina Smillie

I use Coryllos I- IV. However, these classifications are descriptive only, and do not necessarily guide us in either diagnosis or management. The numbers help us describe to another provider how far back under the tongue the membranous portion of the frenulum appears to start. They do not identify how short or tight the frenulum is, nor do they guide our judgment about functional tongue mobility, or give us guidance as to who will, or won't, benefit from frenotomy. Certainly, a baby with an anterior I or II will be easily identified, and just as easily clipped. But if such a long frenulum, all the way to the tip of the tongue, also extends high from the floor of the mouth to the raised tip of the tongue, appearing as a large sail, the baby may be able to lift and extend no problem, and may not actually need the procedure to breastfeed easily and comfortably. Whereas another baby, with what appears to have a shorter and more minor posterior frenulum, may have more dramatically restricted mobility of strong functional consequence. And of course, more commonly, babies with tight Coryllos I ties typically benefit dramatically from revision, whereas stretchy IIIs usually need no intervention at all.

Roberta Martinelli and Irene Marchesan

There are great anatomic variations among lingual frenula. Concerning altered lingual frenula, some are short and others are long. They may be thick or thin. The frenulum attachment to the tongue also varies. Based on these aspects, we classify lingual frenulum as normal, or altered, and when necessary we describe the type of alteration, such as short or long, thick or thin, etc. The restriction of tongue movements is the most important aspect that must be observed because the movements interfere with the functions.

Pamela Douglas

Current definitions of ankyloglossia tend to confuse oral and tongue function (which is affected by multiple variables, and in particular by fit and hold) with structure (which is highly anatomically variable for both the tongue length and appearance, and lingual and maxillary frenula).

Identification of classic tongue-tie

Here, I define CTT as Type 1 and 2 on the Coryllos scale (Watson Genna, 2016). In clinical practice, I also find it useful to rate the anterior membrane by the percentage of the under-surface of the tongue into which the membrane connects, applying the first two categories of the Griffiths Classification System (Griffiths, 2004).

There is a wide spectrum of lingual frenula morphologies and elasticities, and deciding where to draw a line between normal variant, and classic tongue-tie, will depend on clinical judgement concerning the infant's capacity for pain-free efficient milk transfer. If the mother-baby pair are able to breastfeed comfortably with a visible anterior membrane (and many do), then this is not actually a "tie" of the tongue, but merely a visible anterior membrane, requiring no further intervention.

Identification of PTT and ULT

Most unfashionably, I find no use for the diagnoses of PTT and ULT, and argue that they are misconceptions. In my experience, a wide spectrum of normal anatomic lingual and maxillary frenula variants are currently being misdiagnosed as a PTT and ULT. Labial frenula may be classified type I-IV (Kotlow, 2015), but should not be pathologized as "ties," let alone surgically ablated.

Clinical tools merely aid clinical judgment

I've learned, over the years, that clinical tools need to be simple, and only applied as aids in support of our clinical judgment, if we want best outcomes. The skill of the clinician, whether in breastfeeding support or otherwise, is to synthesize a great deal of complex information across multiple domains, and to arrive at a clinical judgment about the likely efficacy or otherwise of intervention. Clinical judgment starts with training, but is built on experience. It is rarely useful (and may be dangerous) to rely on reductionist approaches, including simplistic numerical scales, as a substitute for clinical judgment (Strumberg & Martin, 2016).

For example, although the Hazelbaker Assessment Tool for Lingual Frenulum Function (ATLFF) is a pioneering contribution, bringing us our first systematized approach to examination of the infant's tongue and oral connective tissues, it has been demonstrated to be unreliable as a tool for decision-making concerning frenotomy (Ballard et al., 2002; Madlon-Kay et al., 2008; Ricke et al., 2005). In clinical practice, many of the item criteria are highly subjective and dependent on the infant's interest in cooperating on the day of assessment. Although one study found moderate interrater reliability on the ATLFF's structural items, the authors did not find interrater reliability on most of the functional items (Amir et al., 2006). It became apparent to me that there is no correlation between what the tongue is observed to do during oral examinations and what occurs during breastfeeding, other than in the case of classic tongue-tie. Applying the ATLFF used up precious consultation time that could have gone into clinical breastfeeding support, and I finally abandoned it, creating my own pragmatic assessment tool instead.

References

Amir, L., James, J.P., & Donath, S.M. (2006). Reliability of the Hazelbaker Assessment Tool for Lingual Frenulum Function. *International Breastfeeding Journal*, 1:3.

Ballard, J.L., Auer, C.E., & Khoury, J.C. (2002). Ankyloglossia: Assessment, incidence, and effect of frenuloplasty on the breastfeeding dyad. *Pediatrics*, 110, e63.

De Castro Martinelli, R.L., et al. (2016). Validity and reliability of the neonatal tongue screening test. *Revista CEFAC*, 18(6), 1323-1331.

Greenhalgh, T. (2014). *How to read a paper*, 5th edition. Oxford: John Wiley and Sons, Ltd.

Griffiths, D.M. (2004). Do tongue ties affect breastfeeding? *Journal of Human Lactation*, 20, 411.

Hazelbaker, A.K. (1993). *The assessment tool for lingual frenulum function: use in a lactation consultant private practice.* (Master's thesis. Pacific Oaks College, 1993). Self-published.

Hazelbaker, A. (2010). *Tongue-tie: morphogenesis, impact, assessment and treatment.* Columbus, OH: Aidan and Eva Press.

Kotlow L. (2015). Diagnosing and understanding the maxillary lip-tie (superior labial, the maxillary labial frenum) as it relates to breastfeeding. *Journal of Human Lactation, 29,* 458-464.

Madlon-Kay, D., Ricke, L., Baker, N., & DeFor, T.A. (2008). Case series of 148 tongue-tied newborn babies evaluated with the assessment tool for lingual function. *Midwifery, 24,* 353-357.

Ricke, L., Baker, N., & Madlon-Kay, D. (2005). Newborn tongue-tie: prevalence and effect on breastfeeding. *Journal of American Board of Family Practice, 8,* 1-8.

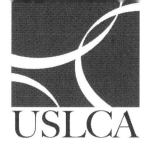

Treating Tongue-Tie

Keywords: tongue-tie, treatment, surgical revision

If a tongue-tie is to be revised, what is the best technique for accomplishing that? There is some debate in the field about whether scissors or laser is most effective. Both techniques seem efficacious. This section also addresses which professionals should be performing the revision. Our panelists represent a wide range of disciplines, so some refer, and others perform the revisions themselves.

What are the Best Techniques for Treating Tongue-Tie?

Catherine Watson Genna

In my experience, scissors work well and are very fast. I also like the control and lack of burning around the incision of the carbon dioxide laser. The skill of the practitioner wielding the tool is more important than which tool is used. That said, laser can more easily divide scar tissue, so is particularly good if a revision is needed.

James Murphy

Iris scissors or laser release are equally effective with similar results. The difference is in the skill of the provider, not the tool used to perform the release.

Christina Smillie

In our area, I prefer scissors, because with the providers in our area who use this technique we see much quicker and better results. Certainly, for simple anterior tongue-ties, I and II, using laser would be like using laser to trim cuticles or get a haircut.

For posterior tongue-ties, I understand the rationale for laser, but it's in the execution where I see problems. With laser by dentists in our area, we see too many babies in pain for extended periods of time, large unnecessarily wide gashes, and a lot of oral aversion. Plus, way too many babies who come to us after a posterior frenotomy with the same breastfeeding problem they had in the first place, which is to say, the intervention did nothing for the baby or the mother. And interestingly, I find that very few dentists are interested in following up, so very few of them seem to be aware of how well or poorly their intervention worked for these families. However, I imagine these procedures are user dependent, and it may be that laser works better in some hands than in others. Certainly, cold laser is supposed to be an improvement, but I have yet to see much difference with the patients in my area. While there are good studies to show the efficacy of revision for anteriors, there are just not yet good studies on any of these interventions for posteriors. So, for the time being, we have to go by our own somewhat subjective and flawed observations.

Roberta Martinelli and Irene Marchesan

In Brazil, frenotomy with divulsion is the most common tongue-tie revision for infants demonstrating excellent results. In children and adults, frenectomy procedure with scissor and scalpel is the most frequent technique.

Martin Kaplan

As a pediatric dentist with experience in tongue-tie treatments from scalpel for older patients, and a trained a laser dental surgeon,

I have an absolute preference for this precise surgical tool. I must point out that a laser is a generic term for the various types that can be used. There are two current types of lasers being used for frenotomy. They are the optic lasers that remove tissue by non-contact ablation and the hot tip diodes that remove tissue with mechanical-thermal contact. This is an important distinction as the lasers perform differently on tissue.

The optic lasers are the CO_2 and Erbium family of lasers. These lasers are highly absorbed by water in the oral mucosa and have very shallow penetration (very important for the thin mucosa of the newborn). They use laser energy to heat up the tissue to 100 degrees Celsius, which is the boiling point of water, and they cause the cells to instantly vaporize. They do this at tissue depths of 20 -50 microns of penetration (for a visual comparison a human hair averages about 120 microns in diameter). So, there is an added safety factor in the surgical precision of the frenulum revision. The diode contact lasers vary in thermal temperature of 500 to 1200 degrees Celsius, and this is the temperature that touches the tissue, and has a deeper heated tissue depth of approximately 2500 microns (2.5 mm.). They are not as accurate and have a smaller window of tissue accuracy.

I have used all classes of lasers mentioned above, and I do have a preference for CO_2. However, I must pause here and say that any well-trained laser surgical provider should be able to adjust his/her technique to compensate for the laser he/she is trained to use for the best clinical results. The organizations that I recommend for laser training are the ALD (Academy of Laser Dentistry), and the ABLS (American Board of Laser Surgery), who have the best science-based guideline for education. This applies for any surgical procedure.

Alison Hazelbaker

Does anybody know the answer to this question? No comparison studies have ever been done.

It is premature to say that one technique over another is superior. We must keep in mind that most studies on tongue-tie revision have used scissors, with excellent results. Any assertion that this or that technique is superior, is based on opinion and, perhaps, comfort level. The exception to the above statements involves lasers. Not every laser is suitable for infant frenectomy due to the physics that govern their functioning (Convissar, 2011; Kaplan, Hazelbaker & Vitruk, 2015; Vitruk, 2014; Vogel & Venugopalan, 2003).

The current trend to do the deeper frenotomy (diamond-shaped wound) with scissors arose, not because of research, but due to a phenomenon called GOBSAT (Good Ole Boys Sitting Around a Table). A Toronto meeting of tongue-tie clinicians, researchers, and surgeons, at which I was present, and at which various aspects of tongue-tie assessment and treatment were discussed, resulted in an informal experiment. One surgeon suggested everyone try the deeper frenotomy because it appeared to be working for his patients. The others were intrigued and said they would try it. Somehow this turned into an edict that all babies should have a deep frenotomy rather than simply cutting back near to the tongue-base without generating a diamond-shaped wound. Laser frenectomy always results in a diamond-shaped wound because it is removal of tissue, rather than an incision into the tissue.

I look forward to carefully controlled comparison studies on surgical techniques and devices. Until then, I will stick to what the evidence shows works, and that has little potential to do harm according to that same evidence.

Pamela Douglas

In order to answer this, we need to consider the biomechanics of infant suck during breastfeeding, including the role of the tongue and its necessary tethering tissues.

The model of infant sucking, upon which laser surgery for PTT and ULT is based, has been shown to be inaccurate by recent ultrasound studies (Douglas & Geddes, 2017; Geddes & Sakalidis, 2016). The upper lip is not involved in breastfeeding or milk transfer, other than to rest neutrally against the breast, and contributes (with multiple other contact sites during the symmetric face-breast bury) towards the seal. It certainly does not need to flange for pain-free milk transfer. Actually, if we can see the upper lip, we are inviting inefficient milk transfer, fussiness at the breast, and nipple pain for many breastfeeding pairs. The tongue does not take an active lead in infant sucking, but responds dynamically to intra-oral breast tissue volume: that is, the tongue's shape, elevation, and spread conform to the amount of breast tissue in the mouth (Douglas & Geddies, 2017; Geddes & Sakalidis, 2016).

The critical biomechanical driver of healthy infant suck is a reflex depression of the jaw, which generates intra-oral vacuum. If the baby is fitted well into the woman's body, this repeated reflex action incrementally draws more and more breast tissue into the mouth until the jaw is held wide open, the nipple tip protected near the junction of the hard and soft palate, and optimal milk transfer occurs. The tongue does not need to actively lift midway to the palate, to lateralize, or to extend beyond the lower gum/ inner edge of lower lip. It does not strip the breast or have peristaltic movements. In fact, the concept of peristalsis has been inappropriately applied to the tongue, since it refers to sequential muscular contractions in a hollow tube. We are describing this new understanding of the biomechanics of infant suck in more detail in a new paper (Douglas & Geddes, 2017).

Since the tongue does not need to actively grip or strip the breast, or compress the breast for milk transfer, but simply follows the jaw depression and molds around the available intra-oral breast tissue volume, we do not need to rely on unproven methods, such as laser surgery, to try to establish increased tongue mobility: a simple scissors frenotomy for a classic tongue-tie allows the tongue to safely perform its molding and cushioning role.

To Whom Do You Refer for Tongue-Tie Revision?

Catherine Watson Genna

I am fortunate to have a number of skilled ear, nose, and throat (ENT) physicians, breastfeeding medicine physicians, and dentists to refer to, depending on the frenulum characteristics, and the family's preference and insurance coverage.

James Murphy

I do the revision.

Martin Kaplan

This question does not apply to me as I am a provider.

Roberta Martinelli and Irene Marchesan

In Brazil, the assessment and diagnosis of tongue-tie is usually performed by SLPs. When there is lingual frenulum alteration, the patient is referred to health professional experienced in tongue-tie revision.

Alison Hazelbaker

Over the 31 years of my practice as an IBCLC, I have developed a wonderful working relationship with a neonatologist in my community. A great deal of trust in his skill has developed after getting excellent results in over 99% of the cases I have sent to him. He uses blunt-ended sterile surgical scissors, and rarely performs a "deep" frenotomy. He stops just before a diamond-shaped wound is generated the vast majority of the time. In all but one case, this approach was sufficient to restore the tongue's optimal range of motion. Of course, I also managed latch and milk supply, and sometimes had to work with the baby's suck, especially when the tongue-tie was only one issue in a plethora of issues, or if the baby was older and had more compensations to correct.

Only one case I sent to him resulted in a need for a second revision. The baby scarred excessively for an unknown reason. The frenotomy had to be repeated once, and then the sucking issue completely resolved. This case was the only case of mine in 31 years for which a re-revision was needed.

Recently, I met with an oral surgeon who has been using CO_2 laser to perform infant frenectomy for many years. Several pediatricians in our large community refer their tongue-tied infant patients to him. He has gotten excellent results, never needs to do a second revision, and does not advocate stretching exercises post-treatment. I have added him to my referral list for those mothers wanting laser revision.

Carmela Baeza

Here in Spain, the impact of tongue-tie on breastfeeding is not well known among health care providers, and therefore it can be quite difficult to find someone willing to revise a tie. Traditionally, in our health care system, it is the pediatric surgeon, or the ENT, who revises tongue-ties. However, since these are specialists, mother needs to get referred to them by the baby's primary care pediatrician. This often becomes an obstacle course. If the primary care pediatrician detects that ankyloglossia is a problem, the baby is referred to the specialist. If the specialist agrees that the tongue-tie is causing problems, he will revise it. This whole referral process may take from two weeks to two months, depending on bureaucratic factors. A typical scenario is when either the pediatrician or the specialist "don't believe in tongue-tie" (often expressed in those terms), or are not willing to refer or treat tongue-tie until it has impacted on speech, or until the child has reached a certain age.

Currently, most lactation consultants here are referring to any local *trained* provider that is known by word of mouth to revise tongue-ties in breastfeeding infants as soon as possible. This may be a pediatrician, surgeon, ENT, odontologist, family physician, or likewise. Often, we've had to create our own networks by suggesting to health care provider colleagues who were personal friends if they would be interested in acquiring the skills for tongue-tie revision so that we could refer our infants to them. This method has worked quite well.

Pamela Douglas

In my view, a severe classic tongue-tie in a newborn should receive a simple scissors frenotomy as soon as possible in order to protect the woman from potential nipple damage. I perform frenotomies with scissors for CTTs in our community setting: all that is necessary to achieve excellent outcomes once intra-oral breast tissue volume is optimized through fit and hold – though the next step is to find funding for studies to investigate this.

Since a simple scissors frenotomy for a classic tongue-tie, or anterior membrane, is pain-free and of minimal risk, I may, with parental consent, err on the side of performing this, even if I'm uncertain about its necessity. In my view, simple scissors frenotomy can be performed by any registered health professional, such as midwife, GP, pediatrician, or lactation consultant with a health professional background, who has received frenotomy training.

A severe CTT that appears at risk of hemorrhage due to vascularized tissues may benefit from laser surgery, which will control the bleeding, but most of us won't encounter these, since they are very rare. I would refer to an ENT surgeon for this, who may use laser.

I can imagine occasions when a clinician might decide, having optimized intra-oral breast tissue volume, that some release of the oral connective tissues might be helpful. In practice, I don't find this necessary other than with CTT, as the critical repair to breastfeeding occurs when intra-oral breast tissue volume is optimized. But even if a clinician decided that this scissors release might be worthwhile, there is no need for a diagnosis. The use of diagnoses increases parental pressure for intervention, even if parents are advised that the diagnosed condition is harmless (Scherer et al., 2013). New diagnoses should only be introduced with great caution, because they risk a cascade of overtreatment (Morgan et al., 2015; Saini et al., 2017).

I no longer refer to pediatric dentists who use scissors, due to the risk of hemorrhage from their deep incisions, having observed babies subjected to painful sutures under the tongue, or in the upper gum, to control bleeding. Laser surgery reduces the risk of hemorrhage, but the studies used to claim that laser surgery for PTT or ULT improves breastfeeding outcomes show substantial bias, and should be viewed with great skepticism (Douglas, 2017a, 2017b). Standards of evidence need to be high to demonstrate outcomes: why do our mothers and babies deserve a vastly poorer quality of science compared to, say, patients with diabetes or osteoarthritis? Why should they be subjected to the inevitable risk of unintended outcomes that arise when simplistic "quick-fix" interventions are put into complex systems? (Douglas, 2016, 2017b; Francis et al., 2015; Power & Murphy, 2015; Reid & Rajput, 2014).

Christina Smillie

As a pediatrician, I do the simple anterior frenuli myself, Coryllos classifications I-III, if restricted lingual mobility warrants it. For those that appear to be submucosal (Coryllos IV), or those Coryllos I-III that I have snipped that I think deserve further revision, I refer primarily to an excellent pediatric ENT group in our area. This is a group who understand how the infant oral structures work while breastfeeding, independently evaluate for lingual mobility, and make their own judgements: they don't think that every referral demands revision. That is to say, while they usually agree with me, they don't rubber stamp. I like this in any specialist I refer to. There is one dentist in our area who also makes careful assessments before deciding for himself whether laser is indicated.

However, there are many dentists in our area who will laser any baby who is brought to their office, willing to take anyone else's word for it, because they know nothing about breastfeeding or lactation, or worse, they have learned just enough to be quite certain that every common infant or breastfeeding problem is a sign of tongue-tie. I imagine choice of consultants will vary from geographic area to area, depending on the skill, expertise, and professionalism of the different providers, which may well be more important than their particular discipline. I am suspicious of those who are big on self-promotion.

References

Convissar, R. (2011). *Principles and Practice of Laser Dentistry*. St. Louis, MO: Mosby Elsevier.

Douglas, P.S. (2016, under review). Why Ghaheri et al's 2016 study does not show that surgical release for the diagnoses of posterior tongue-tie and upper lip-tie improve breastfeeding outcomes.

Douglas, P.S. (2017b, under review). Making sense of studies which claim benefits of frenotomy in the absence of classic tongue-tie.

Douglas, P.S., & Geddes, D.B. (2017, final stages). Practice-based interpretation of ultrasound studies leads the way to less pharmaceutical and surgical intervention for breastfeeding babies and more effective clinical support.

Francis, D.O., Krishnaswami, S., & McPheeters, M. (2015). Treatment of ankyloglossia and breastfeeding outcomes: A systematic review. *Pediatrics*, *135*(6), e1467-e1474.

Geddes, D.T., & Sakalidis, V.S. (2016). Ultrasound imaging of breastfeeding - a window to the inside: methodology, normal appearances, and application. *Journal of Human Lactation*, Doi:10.1177/0890334415626152.

Kaplan, M., Hazelbaker, A.K., & Vitruk, P. (2015). Infant frenectomy with 10,600 nm dental CO_2 laser. *WAGD Newsletter, April*.

Morgan, D.J., Brownless, S.B., Leppin, A.L., Kressin, N., Dhruva, S.S., Levin, L. et al. (2015). Setting a research agenda for medical overuse. *BMJ, 351*, h4534.

Power, R., & Murphy, J. (2015). Tongue-tie and frenotomy in infants with breastfeeding difficulties: achieving a balance. *Archives of Disease in Childhood, 100*, 489-494.

Reid, N., & Rajput, N. (2014). Acute feed refusal followed by Staphylococcus aureus wound infection after tongue-tie release. *Journal of Paediatrics and Child Health, 50*, 1030-1031.

Saini, V., Brownlee, S., Elshaug, A.G., Glasziou, P., & Iona Health. (2017). Addressing overuse and underuse around the world. *The Lancet*. Retrieved from: http://dx.doi.org/10.1016/50140-6736(16)32753-9.

Vitruk, P. (2014). Oral soft tissue laser ablative & coagulation efficiencies spectra. *Implant Practice US*, November.

Vogel, A., & Venugopalan, V. (2003). Mechanisms of pulsed laser ablation of biological tissues. *Chemical Review, 103*(2), 577-644.

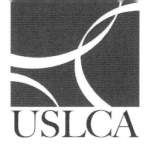

Clinical
Photos

Roberta Martinelli

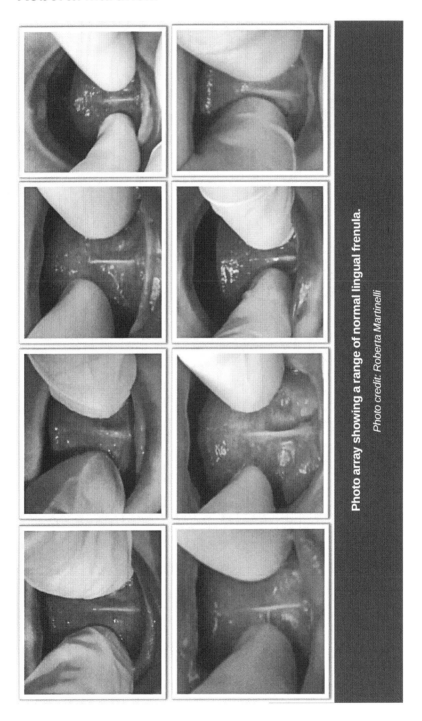

Photo array showing a range of normal lingual frenula.
Photo credit: Roberta Martinelli

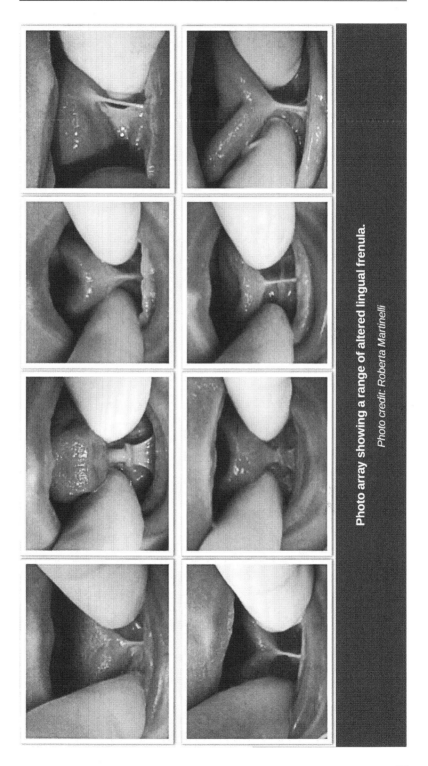

Photo array showing a range of altered lingual frenula.
Photo credit: Roberta Martinelli

Catherine Watson Genna

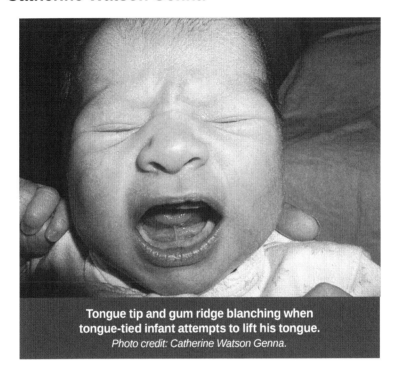

Tongue tip and gum ridge blanching when tongue-tied infant attempts to lift his tongue.
Photo credit: Catherine Watson Genna.

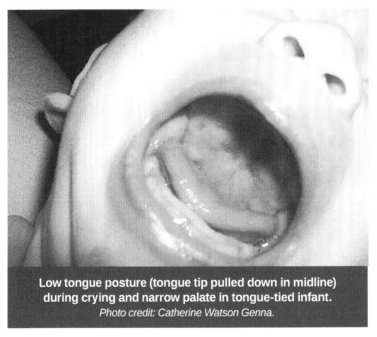

Low tongue posture (tongue tip pulled down in midline) during crying and narrow palate in tongue-tied infant.
Photo credit: Catherine Watson Genna.

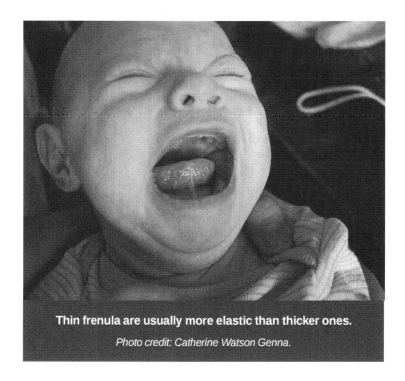

Thin frenula are usually more elastic than thicker ones.

Photo credit: Catherine Watson Genna.

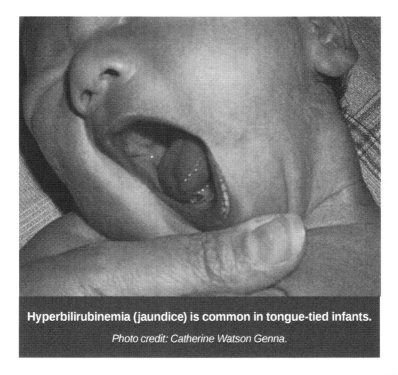

Hyperbilirubinemia (jaundice) is common in tongue-tied infants.

Photo credit: Catherine Watson Genna.

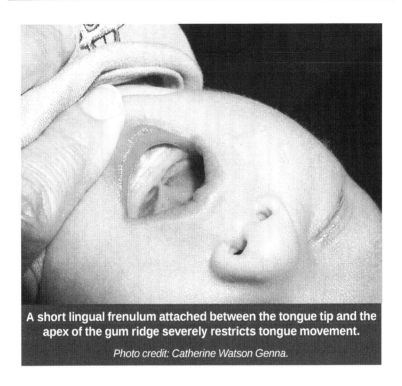

A short lingual frenulum attached between the tongue tip and the apex of the gum ridge severely restricts tongue movement.

Photo credit: Catherine Watson Genna.

Carmela Baeza

This is a 28-day-old infant who came to my practice for an urgent consultation: she was refusing to latch. A frenotomy had been done 48 hours before. She was failng to thrive. It was an anterior tongue-tie, but after revising it, the surgeon decided to go deeper because he thought there was also a posterior tie. He used scissors, and cauterized the wound with silver nitrate.

When I saw the baby, she had barely eaten for 48 hours. After she refused the breast a few times, mother expressed some milk and had been able to feed her child with a bottle, although she described it as a battle.

As you can see in the image, the revision area is covered with silver nitrate (black) and around it is a hypertrophic scar tissue reaction (white). The baby's upper lip is swollen. And the baby is desperate.

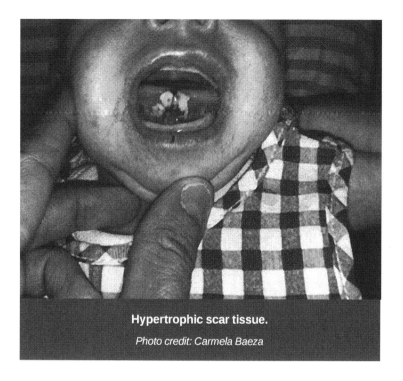

Hypertrophic scar tissue.
Photo credit: Carmela Baeza

The intervention was to gently wash the nitrate off with 0.9% saline solution, give the baby an oral dose of ibuprofen, and feed her expressed breast milk. For 12 hours, she only tolerated syringe feeding (not finger feeding or cup feeding). After that she went back to the breast, although her suck was not comfortable and effective until three days later. The failure to thrive for which she had been diagnosed, and ankyloglossia, were resolved two weeks later.

The take-aways from this case are: 1. for frenotomies, choose a professional who knows what he or she is doing, and who is gentle while doing it. 2. Revising a posterior tongue-tie is not a simple snip. It is a painful intervention for the infant that may have negative effects on short-term breastfeeding. It is imperative that only infants who have been *correctly diagnosed* as having a restricted tongue movement due to a posterior ankyloglossia be subjected to these procedures.

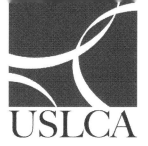

Post-Revision Instructions and Pain Relief

Keywords: tongue-tie, infants, breastfeeding, post-revision care

What should parents do after their babies' tongue-ties have been revised? This is one of the most-contentious issues when considering tongue-tie. Our panelists differ in their recommendations, and this section shows the range of views. This section also includes recommendations regarding pain relief.

Do Babies Need Post-Revision Stretching of the Wound Site?

Christina Smillie

No. Definitely not, with the anterior snips. With the posterior snips, my anecdotal observation is that stretching and pressure is one of the causes of oral aversion, and probably slows healing. I don't see the need for it since babies are super oriented to their tongues, and stretch and use their tongues a LOT, quite naturally, with every feed and oral expression (i.e., all the time). The size of the tongue on the neurocortical homunculus should give us a clue. Plus, ordinary wound care teaches us that we delay healing by messing around pressing on wounded tissue. The fact that the babies react to these exercises with pain is another clue that we shouldn't be doing it.

Babies heal very fast from any wound, injury, or incision, and we don't need to do any such care with any of our other surgical interventions. We do not pull on pierced ears, or tug on poor little guys' circumcised glans. Nor do we pull and stretch women's abdominal incisions after a C-section. That makes zero sense from a wound-healing point of view. Some folks are telling families to do these exercises multiple times a day for weeks, when babies' tissues are fully healed, in a much shorter time than that. Gentle massage for a few days might be helpful if it promotes good blood flow and the baby enjoys the game. One of our ear, nose, and throat (ENT) specialists sometimes suggests these, but briefly. The other, his partner, never does, and I don't see any difference.

For myself, I was doing anterior revisions for several years before anyone ever talked about exercises. So then, for awhile, I started suggesting the parents use fingers to encourage the baby to lift tongue, with no touch involved. However, I only do those thin membranous anteriors, and after awhile, I just didn't see the physiologic point and abandoned the practice. We have NO studies on this.

Catherine Watson Genna

I wish we knew the answer to this. I have seen infants who really needed the tongue to be lifted several times a day to prevent scarring, and others who healed beautifully with nothing but continued breastfeeding. There are some hints in the research (O'Callahan's case series, for example) that fewer revisions are needed when the tongue is elevated to stretch the wound. I think the most important thing is that if exercises are done, they are done respectfully and as gently as possible, to avoid pain and stress to the baby and family.

James Murphy

Some infants do well with good breastfeeding alone following tongue-tie release, but the majority need to perform wound stretching to achieve an acceptable final result. I believe the final result with stretching is superior to nursing alone.

Alison Hazelbaker

This strategy also arose out of Good Olde Boys Sitting Around a Table (GOBSAT). The wound-healing science entered the discussion only recently. When contemplating this question, several issues come to my mind:

» If, up to now, we garnered excellent results for breast-feeding without performing the deep frenotomy, AND no other stretching was required other than normal tongue movements performed during tongue play and feeding, why are we advocating these strategies now?

» If we garnered excellent results without doing the diamond-shaped, and the diamond-shaped wound *requires* more aggressive treatment for "proper" wound healing, then doesn't performing the deep frenotomy generate an avoidable iatrogenic problem?

» These wound "healing" strategies are untested, and are therefore experimental. These experiments are being performed on the most vulnerable population: our babies.

» Three issues have arisen from using these strategies that are anecdotal, but are appearing more and more frequently in discussions: 1. Breast refusal, 2. Parental non-compliance because babies adversely react to the protocols, and 3. Excessive scar tissue formation requiring a repeat procedure.

» Everyone seems to have their own protocol, many claiming that their protocol is the best. Which protocol would be best if a protocol of stretching would be warranted?

» Claims are being made that it is parental non-compliance that causes excessive scar tissue formation requiring repeat revision, BUT the wound-healing science shows that it is excessive manipulation of the wound that causes excessive scar tissue formation (Desmouliere, Darby, & Gabbiani, 2003; Darby, Laverdet, Bonte, & Desmouliere, 2014; Gabbiani, 2004; Li & Wang, 2011; Tomasek et al., 2002). At what point do we use the science as our guide?

Wound contracture is part of the normal wound-healing process. The science shows that some organic movement near a wound to signal the tissue to heal in ways that best allow for that organic movement results in better wound healing (Darby, Laverdet, Bonte, & Desmouliere, 2014; Gabbiani, 2004). The science also shows that excessive disturbance of the wound causes prolonged healing and denser scar tissue formation to stabilize the area (Darby, Laverdet, Bonte, & Desmouliere, 2014). When has a health professional ever recommended wound manipulation for proper surgical wound healing on any other part of the body other than normal body movements?

In the case of tongue-tie, keeping the tongue moving *without disturbing* the normal course of wound healing makes sense. So in the case of revision wound healing, less may be more when it comes to these post-revision stretches.

Perhaps the best result will be garnered when we use the extensive wound-healing science to help us find the "sweet spot."

Martin Kaplan

This is currently a subject of passionate controversy. The potential for reattachment issue is the touchstone for stretching and post-op care, or AWM (active wound management). This can be caused by multiple factors, such as individual healing differences, physical restrictions due to undiagnosed birth trauma, or in utero positioning (this is where body work is an important component).

I was initially instructed, in my early lectures and seminars, to provide stretching over the wound site to prevent scarring and reattachment. This always bothered me because stretching the edges of a new wound, and rubbing through the center of a fresh surgical site, is counter intuitive. This is very uncomfortable for both the baby and mother, who are already stressed. I decided to adjust my post-op instructions for my parents that were at least less traumatic to the treated tissue. I initiated a glide with an index finger pad (moistened with breastmilk or formula) over the site released. This was much easier for the parents, and less traumatic for the infant.

Since I incorporated CO_2 lasers as a better surgical procedure, I have adjusted my instructions for post-op tongue treatment to incorporate stimulated tongue mobility exercises for extension, lateralization, and grooving of the tongue. This is a much easier process for the parents to accomplish, and much less stressful. Many IBCLCs have used similar exercises to establish better tongue mobility for newborns. Since I have instituted this change, I have noted no increase for needs of revision, in my practice, which currently stands at a proximately 2% to 3%.

Pamela Douglas

Wound stretching places babies at risk of oral aversion, due to repeated uncomfortable or painful digital intrusion. There is no scientific reason to believe that wound stretching post-laser frenotomy alters the inevitable contraction of scar tissue over time. Unfortunately, I regularly see short, thick, white cords of scar tissue under baby's tongues these days, a few months post-frenotomy.

Roberta Martinelli and Irene Marchesan

Tongue movement during breastfeeding is a good frenulum exercise after a revision. For children and adults, we recommend movements of elevation and lateralization of the tongue during the first week after the revision to avoid having the tongue remaining down-positioned (on the floor of the mouth). The patients should be followed up once a week during the first month after a revision for recovery observation. Usually the movements performed by the tongue during the normal functions are sufficient exercises.

What Do You Recommend for Pain Relief During and Following Revision Procedures?

Alison Hazelbaker

The physician to whom I send for scissors frenotomy uses hemostats to gently compress the lingual frenulum. He thinks this may reduce the amount of bleeding and pain the baby experiences during and post procedure. I have mixed feeling about the use of pain relief during the procedure. Numbing agent may make it harder for the baby to go to breast and suck directly after. However, if a hot-tip laser, like diode laser, is used, the hot-tip burns the tissue, potentially causing significant pain. Perhaps pain relief during this procedure would be helpful.

Post procedure, our surgeon recommends some Tylenol for soreness, perhaps one to two doses. We suggest arnica homeopathic for those parents who use alternatives.

Carmela Baeza

I don't do frenotomies, so if you refer to pain relief during the procedure, I cannot answer. However, I have received babies who refuse to nurse, or have an altered sucking pattern, after a frenotomy, especially the more aggressive interventions for "posterior" tongue-tie. In this case, I usually prescribe (as an MD, not as an IBCLC) acetaminophen at an adequate pediatric dose, or if there is important swelling, ibuprofen, for a couple of days. We also work on finding the most comfortable way for these infants to be fed until the breast is comfortable for them again.

James Murphy

For those of us who have had great success releasing tongue and lip ties with iris scissors, a topical anesthetic has been exceedingly safe and effective, although lidocaine with epinephrine really helps with lip frenum anesthesia and elimination of bleeding. Although I would love to purchase a CO_2 laser ($32,000–$100,000), that would be a financial disaster. Hence, LMX4 and EMLA are very useful, safe, and effective. Dr. Ghaheri, and some local dentists, use a higher concentration of lidocaine, prilocaine, and tetracaine very safely for their releases. Use a small amount only at the operative site.

References

Darby, I. A., Laverdet, B., Bonté, F., & Desmoulière, A. (2014). Fibroblasts and myofibroblasts in wound healing. *Clinical, Cosmetic and Investigational Dermatology, 7*, 301–311.

Desmoulière, A., Darby, I. A., & Gabbiani, G. (2003). Normal and pathologic soft tissue remodeling: Role of the myofibroblast, with special emphasis on liver and kidney fibrosis. *Laboratory Investigation, 83*, 1689–1707.

Gabbiani, G. (2004). The evolution of the myofibroblast concept: A key cell for wound healing and fibrotic disease. *Giornale di Gerontologia, 52*, 280–282.

Li, B., & Wang, J. (2011). Fibroblasts and myofibroblasts in wound healing: Force generation and measurement. *Journal of Tissue Viability, 20*(4), 108–120.

Tomasek, J. J., Gabbiani, G., Hinz, B., Chaponnier, C., & Brown, R. A. (2002). Myofibroblasts and mechano-regulation of connective tissue remodelling. *Nature Reviews. Molecular Cellular Biology, 3*(5), 349–363.

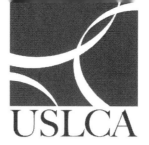

USLCA

Posterior Tie

Keywords: posterior tongue-tie; breastfeeding; identification; treatment

Posterior tongue-tie is another controversial topic in the tongue-tie world. A posterior tongue-tie is a class-IV tongue-tie. It may be submucosal (i.e., underneath the mucous membrane covering). Babies with this kind of tie are often misidentified as having a short tongue. Revision is more involved, and there is disagreement about whether this condition exists, and to what extent. Our panelists weigh in on this topic.

Does Posterior Tongue-Tie Exist?

Carmela Baeza

My thoughts are that it is not a clear, single entity, like anterior tongue-tie. It is a restriction of tongue movement, certainly, but this tissue restriction can be because of various factors: inelasticity of the tissue itself or lack of functional movement because of tensions in the area. There can also be impacts on other structures, such as the cranial nerves, which would alter not only tongue movement but also sensory input. Restricted tongue movement requires a lot of clinical observation and thought.... And some infants have restrained or altered tongue movements, and we just can't figure out why. Blaming a single entity like "posterior tongue-tie" is oversimplistic (See Figure below).

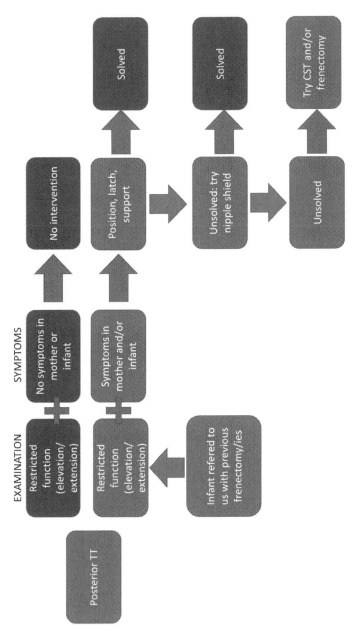

Algorithm for assessing the posterior tie. Carmela Baeza, MD, IBCLC.

Catherine Watson Genna

Since I'm a member of the team that coined the phrase, I certainly think it exists. Again, it's important to differentiate between a normal frenulum attached along the mid to posterior tongue versus an inelastic frenulum in the same place. Roberta Martinelli and Irene Marchesan (PhD speech pathologists and participants in this round table) examined the tissue structure of restrictive frenula and found that they were histologically altered.

James Murphy

·I prefer to call this a submucosal tongue-tie as that is more descriptive. I always find a submucosal fibrous band behind every "anterior" sail membrane. Most of my patients have a submucosal tie only. Pediatricians are getting much better at recognizing the sail membranes, and releasing them, which improves the overall breastfeeding situation but often does not resolve the problem.

Alison K. Hazelbaker

Do you mean to ask about any frenum whose ventral tongue attachment is behind the tongue body-blade juncture or "submucosal tie?" The tendency to say posterior tie when what is meant is "submucosal tie" muddies the discussion waters. There are truly tongue-tied babies who have a ventral tongue attachment of the lingual frenum behind the body-blade juncture. According to the Todd prevalence data, these comprise the smaller number of tongue-ties, accounting for only 30% of the total number of ties in his cohort. I would like to see more research done to either confirm or flesh out his data.

I have always had concerns about the proposed "submucosal" tongue-tie category. A few years before Catherine Watson Genna started speaking about her "submucosal tie" theory, I was intensively using craniosacral therapy as an adjunct to lactation management to help resolve biomechanically based infant sucking issues, with excellent results. I did a pilot study that showed a significant difference in suck-swallow-breathe coordination as measured by the Neonatal Oral-Motor Assessment Scale (NOMAS) before and after a series of craniosacral treatments. I never submitted the study for publication because I was in the middle of my doctoral program. The babies whom I was treating with craniosacral therapy presented with similar characteristics as Watson Genna's baby clients whom she described as having submucosal tongue-ties.

It appears that we were both observing tongue "restrictions," but attributing them to different etiologies.

After hearing Watson Genna present on the subject, I started to correlate the ATLFF and NOMAS scores with Watson Genna's description of "sub-mucosal tie" in babies presenting at my clinic. These babies routinely scored borderline on the ATLFF and dysfunctional on the NOMAS: they had the appearance characteristics of the sub-mucosal tie as described in the Coryllos classification schema, but the function of a biomechanically based sucking problem. This led me to coin the term "faux tie" to categorize these babies.

Tongue-tie is a congenital anomaly that occurs because of a failure in development. Tongue-tie is, therefore, a malformation. Faux tie, on the other hand, is acquired rather than congenital. Faux ties are biomechanical sucking issues that are caused by soft-tissue restrictions, or injury and/or cranial nerve, compromise thereby changing tongue posture. The change in tongue posture causes the tongue underside and mouth floor to tighten, in turn causing tongue movement restriction. Often the lingual frenum becomes tight as well, mimicking a true tie (Hazelbaker, 2010).

Future research is needed to elucidate the following:

» Is sub-mucosal tie, as per Coryllos and Watson Genna, an actual form of the congenital anomaly we call tongue-tie?

» When the characteristics of sub-mucosal tie are present, does the condition respond to therapy, surgery, both, or neither?

» Which approach best restores proper suck-swallow-breathe coordination without doing harm?

» How do we clearly delineate tongue-tie from other tongue-restrictions and anomalies?

Because we are paying better attention to the role that tongue-movement deficits play in breastfeeding problems, we are paying better attention to the role that tongue movement deficits play in breastfeeding problems, we have a unique opportunity to identify all the various causes of those deficits. Tongue-tie is only one causal factor. I look forward to continuing respectful dialectic and research that will help us delineate those causes and prepare us better to formulate and implement effective solutions.

Martin Kaplan

I think the current controversy is because only anterior tongue-tie (the classical tie) was recognized and just quickly released with a scissors.

There are some physicians that just thought that tongue-ties do not exist or they will stretch out or tear on their own. Others would just introduce formula or reflux meds because the baby was a poor "nurser," or had true reflux. (I see and hear this much too often.)

When I first began treating newborns, I did not understand the big deal about the differentiation between tongue-tie types. I thought, "a tongue-tie is a tongue-tie." However, there obviously are different presentations, and they do not all look the same, feel the same, nor function the same. I see anterior ties and posterior ties. You can even break these posterior ties down to where the frenum is located, and how it affects elevation, lateralization, and grooving. There can be tongue humping, lack of cupping, spread, and posterior dimpling, which all present with various signs, including the inability to lift up the head properly. Or it presents as the baby sleeping with an arched back head (as if he is positioning himself for baby CPR position for obtaining an open airway).

When you can identify that there are different presentations, then you can even identify the various types of tissue presentation, such as corded, hourglass, Eiffel tower, thin, thick, wide, fleshy, or fibrous. These all give an indication of what to expect when one treated the frenum. When you have these presentations identified, you can better adjust your laser treatments for the tissue type. If you use a scissors or scalpel, and there is significant bleeding, then you cannot easily identify the entirety of the release due to blood-compromised vision. If you are only releasing a thin membrane, then bleeding is not an issue.

As an aside, I believe all releases should be performed in a well-lighted and magnified environment. Vision is very important as to identifying your end of surgery site.

There is also the controversial submucosal tie. This can be called a deep posterior tie. However, I can attest, by my own experience, that there are cases where these types do not present with the usual fibrous restriction. There is more of a wide and tight membrane, which was easily released with laser. Bladed surgery cannot be that exact without involving muscle in the release. This is unnecessary.

Christina Smillie

As stated above, this is a new diagnosis, not yet well-studied, that we need to take care with. Although we don't have the data yet to inform our decisions, families are still walking in the door with problems that require our help, issues that might or might not be attributable to restricted posterior tongue mobility. As a doctor who is also a lactation consultant, I will make the very unfair and gross generalization that while doctors tend to underdiagnose this issue (although more and more pediatricians in my area are actually recognizing posterior tongue-tie as a problem and referring to us), many LCs, just as unfortunately, tend to over diagnose posterior tongue-tie, both too frequently, and way too early. While there are good data to show us that babies with ANTERIOR tongue-ties benefit by treatment, the earlier the better, there is not data to support translating this recommendation to posteriors. And that leap is problematic, precisely because the diagnosis is trickier, and more likely to be wrong. Quick treatment of a false posterior only delays appropriate treatment of what the real problem was.

Roberta Martinelli and Irene Marchesan

The posterior tongue-tie is sometimes referred to as a submucosal tongue-tie. We conducted a study aimed to verify the occurrence of posterior lingual frenulum in infants, and its interference with sucking and swallowing during breastfeeding.

The study included 1,084 newborns who were assessed at 30 days of life, using the Lingual Frenulum Protocol for Infants. Of the 1,084 newborns, 479 (44.2%) had normal lingual frenulum, 380 (35%) had posterior lingual frenulum, and 225 (20.8%) had lingual frenulum alterations. Infants with posterior lingual frenulum did not have any restriction of tongue movement during sucking and swallowing. The occurrence of posterior frenulum in this sample was 35%. The posterior frenulum did not interfere with sucking and swallowing during breastfeeding. Therefore, surgery was not recommended for this sample.

Reference

Hazelbaker, A. (2010). *Tongue-tie: Morphogenesis, impact, assessment and treatment.* Columbus, OH: Aidan and Eva Press.

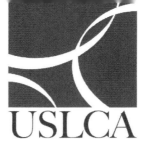

Complementary Techniques to Address Tongue-Tie

Keywords: tongue-tie; torticollis; complementary treatments; craniosacral therapy; physical therapy; chiropractic

Do parents have any alternatives to surgery for addressing tongue-tie? Our panelists agree that latch issues should be assessed first. Other modalities include physical therapy, speech therapy, chiropractic, and craniosacral therapy. In addition, infants should be assessed for other issues, such as torticollis, that may co-occur with tongue-tie. For some parents, complementary techniques may be all that they need to address tongue-tie–related issues. For other parents, surgical release will still be necessary.

Can Complementary Techniques Be Used to Treat Tongue-Tie? How Do You Decide?

Catherine Watson Genna

Basic lactation assistance (optimizing positioning and latch) should always be tried first. If the baby is unable to latch, or causes mother significant pain after a lactation consultation, and there is a clearly restrictive frenulum and no confounders,

I refer. If there is torticollis, physical therapy can help, and speech therapy for weakness of tongue or oral muscles. I also refer to an osteopathic physician who specializes in manipulative medicine for breastfeeding difficulties, several occupational therapists and infant chiropractors who use craniosacral therapy as one of their modalities.

James Murphy

While many body workers claim superior results from body work alone, in my experience, body work is an adjunct to surgical release, and may begin shortly before it, or begin at any time after surgical release. I do not advocate for body work alone when the above criteria for diagnosis of a tongue-tie are met.

Martin Kaplan

Yes, if it is available. It should also be part of the routine comprehensive body evaluation. The concerns here, for me, are that there may be a physical restriction, whether musculoskeletal or fascia tension, that has not been identified for corrective treatment. Form and function are intimately related. If there is a body injury or restriction that the craniosacral therapist (CST) or infant chiropractor determines for treatment, then the physical correction performed body will assist in retaining a surgically necessary intervention.

Position of latch, and ability to improve latch, is huge. This is where an IBCLC, or other trained breast- or bottle-feeding specialist is hugely important. A factor that many surgical providers may not consider in the total care is maternal breast-anatomy problems affecting latch, or there may have been previous breast surgery or chest traumas that affect the ability to produce milk. There may be a psychological component to breastfeeding. There may have been emotional abuse, rape or incest, and the ability of the mother to feel comfortable with this intimate contact cannot be sustained. A team of educated infant and mother-dyad providers is necessary.

I decide by having the mother complete a comprehensive mother-and-baby symptom intake form. This includes the history of term (early/full or late), vaginal or cesarean section delivery, whether hospital or home birth, drug-induced delivery, breast milk letdown issues, who evaluated the baby, and mother nursing. We need to assure that there are no cases treated by visual assessment only. Not every presentation of frenum requires treatment. (See pp. 132–138 for intake protocols.)

Alison K. Hazelbaker

Proper management always takes precedence over surgery and should be the first line of intervention. Proper management includes using evidence-based assessment to garner an accurate diagnosis alongside of typical lactation management strategies, such as positioning and attachment technique. In my experience of using the Assessment Tool for Lingual Frenulum Function (ATLFF) over a 28-year period, scores do not significantly improve with nonsurgical lactation management when a baby is *truly* tongue-tied. The baby may become a better compensator, but actual tongue function does not normalize.

I decide what to do only after taking a thorough history, watching the baby feed, examining the baby, and by using a differential diagnosis process. If the baby has a borderline score on the ATLFF, and has other signs of a biomechanically based sucking issue, I use lactation management strategies in conjunction with craniosacral therapy. I sometimes refer to an occupational therapist (OT) and a chiropractor for optimal results.

Craniosacral therapy (the practice of which is the same as osteopathy as practiced in countries other than the United States) does not resolve a true-tie. But mounting evidence demonstrates its effectiveness in resolving or mitigating biomechanically based sucking issues (Frymann, 1966; Herzhaft-Le Roy, Xhignesse, & Gaboury, 2017; Lund et al., 2011; Maxwell, Fraval, & Osteo, 1998; Pizzolorusso et al., 2013). I am performing research with several colleagues in the UK, and planning research here in the U.S., to further examine the role craniosacral therapy/osteopathy plays in resolving biomechanically based sucking issues.

Can craniosacral therapy/osteopathy be utilized successfully as an adjunct to surgery for tongue-tie? Anecdotally, we see good to excellent results. Formal research will provide more information upon which to base our clinical decisions in regard to this bodywork modality.

One may claim that a double standard exists. Why is it OK to use craniosacral therapy experimentally, and not OK to experiment with surgical remedies? A simple risk assessment answers the question. In the case of torticollis, or plagiocephaly-derived sucking issues, an OT and/or PT *must* be a member of the team. These practitioners have the specialized knowledge and skills needed to quickly and effectively address these significant structural problems.

Carmela Baeza

The correct diagnosis and management of ankyloglossia in the breastfeeding dyad is mainly based, in my opinion, on clinical experience. There are certain types of tongue restriction on which the current assessment tools just don't shed enough light. At the end of the day, management is a judgement call based on the lactation consultant's experience.

This is the reasoning model that I (and the colleagues I work with) use, based on our knowledge and experience (and which will hopefully get more effective as we gain more knowledge and experience).

1. Anterior tongue-ties that do not limit function, and do not impact on mother (no nipple discomfort or pain, obstructions, etc.), nor on infant (no weight-gain issues). I do not intervene.

2. Anterior tongue-ties that impact on mother (nipple discomfort or pain, obstructions, etc.) and/or infant (weight-gain issues), and that *do not* resolve with basic breastfeeding interventions (positioning, latch). Refer for revision. In a group of 68 dyads with these characteristic in the last year at my practice, 100% had great improvement after revision.

3. No visible anterior tongue-tie; when I explore, baby tongue movement is limited (elevation and/or extension and/or lateralization), but there is no impact on mother (no nipple discomfort or pain, obstructions, etc.), nor on infant (no weight-gain issues). I do not intervene.

4. No visible anterior tongue-tie; when I explore, baby tongue movement is limited (elevation and/or extension and/or lateralization), and there is an impact on mother (nipple discomfort or pain, obstructions, etc.), and/or infant (weight-gain issues). We work with different positioning and latch techniques, and very frequently the problem is resolved.

5. No visible anterior tongue-tie; when I explore baby tongue movement is limited (elevation and/or extension and/or lateralization), and there is an impact on mother (nipple discomfort or pain, obstructions, etc.), and/or infant (weight-gain issues). Positioning and latch techniques do

not work. I try nipple shields, if mother is willing. They work fairly often in these cases, although, of course, we have to make sure milk transfer is not diminished.

6. No visible anterior tongue-tie; when I explore, baby tongue movement is limited (elevation and/or extension and/or lateralization), and there is an impact on mother (nipple discomfort or pain, obstructions, etc.), and/or infant (weight-gain issues). Positioning and latch techniques do not work, nipple shields do not work, and this is where it gets murky. My next step is to refer for bodywork (craniosacral, osteopath, speech therapist; my referral is based on the provider's experience rather than the actual field of specialization). Some infants get better, some don't. Other infants I refer for posterior tongue-tie revision. This decision I make based almost solely on clinical experience: after revision, some improve, some don't (60% improve, according to data from our practice). And the few that don't improve after all these interventions are the dramatic cases where all our skills and all the referrals just are not enough. Sometimes these dyads will get better as time goes by, and I am never quite sure which of the interventions did the job, or if it was the time and the support. Sadly, others will partially or totally wean despite our efforts.

Christina Smillie

Definitely. Except for really obvious anterior frenuli, I am very reluctant to "diagnose" tongue-tie on the first visit. Anything that pulls on that hyoid bone has the potential to restrict tongue mobility. And restricted jaw mobility can also interfere with easy tongue mobility. Yes, a baby can have a very tight jaw as the result of restricted tongue mobility, but more often it appears to me that a tight jaw is more likely the cause of what only appears to be restricted tongue mobility. So what looks like a posterior tongue-tie often disappears after a session, or three, with someone truly skilled in craniosacral therapy. Similarly, a baby with frank or subtle torticollis can have restricted tongue mobility, and the pseudo tongue-tie disappears when the torticollis is treated.

Plus, the word tongue is misleadingly simplistic: The tongue is a whole group of interconnected muscles, so the orolingual exam can change dramatically from moment to moment, depending on the baby's state, wakeful or sleepy, hunger or satiety, and so forth, as well as from day to day, depending on tone, on how well nourished or underweight, and so forth. Not that the tongue's anatomy actually changes, but the exam changes because the baby uses the tongue's muscles differently under different circumstances. I find my own very careful exam can look quite different, not just from visit to visit, but even from the beginning of a 2-hour appointment to the end of that same appointment.

Furthermore, a baby who is underweight may conserve energy, and limit his or her tongue use to "drinking at the water fountain," only moving slightly, and only with high milk flow, making it look like he has restricted tongue mobility, whereas once his weight has caught up, he may use his tongue just fine, even on a soft breast and slow flow at the end of a feed. So whereas some professionals may see restricted tongue mobility as the cause of slow weight gain, I often view that apparently limited mobility to be the possible result of the underweight infant's low energy. When this is the case, the apparent posterior tongue-tie can magically disappear *after* we help the baby catch up on his weight and energy by offering him increased calories via a high-flow feeding method.

How do I decide? Primum non nocere. First do no harm. Simple anteriors involve snipping a thin little membrane, simple to diagnose and simple to treat, no negative outcomes to worry about. I'll do those the same day I see them, the sooner the better, if parents are prepared for and want it done. But with posteriors, we need to be careful, because history, exam, diagnosis, and management are ALL tricky. And for such intervention in a baby, we need to be sure the punishment fits the crime. The exam can change so much with the baby's level of activity, it needs to be repeated a couple times; the differential diagnosis is significant, including a lot of chicken-or-egg questions; and there are usually plenty of good rational management options that should be tried first.

Even when a first exam fairly strongly suggests restricted tongue mobility, which might be caused by a submucosal or posterior restriction of the tongue, I will first do whatever else the history and physical suggests might be primary, and give it typically at least a week with other obvious and more benign interventions before jumping to any conclusions. Particularly since this whole diagnosis of posterior tongue-tie is only a dozen years old, and we have yet to see good studies that help guide us as to what signs or symptoms can best predict who will do well by intervention and who won't.

Roberta Martinelli and Irene Marchesan

These techniques are not usual in Brazil. Some health professionals indicate several breastfeeding maneuvers to avoid early weaning and the revision.

Pamela Douglas

This is, in my view, *the* most important question!

The promotion of surgical release of tongue-tie (PTT) and upper lip-tie (ULT) is the latest in a series of inappropriately medicalized interventions for breastfeeding problems (Douglas, 2012, 2013). We inhabit complex biophysical and sociocultural contexts, where "trusting instinct" is definitely not enough for many. The painstaking art and science of supporting a woman and her baby's competence is easily sacrificed to the seduction of the medicalized silver bullet.

Fussing at the breast, difficulty latching, pulling or slipping off, back-arching (signs of positional instability and poor fit and hold), and/or excessive flatus, explosive frothy stools (signs of functional lactose overload) have been mistakenly diagnosed as signs of gastroesophageal reflux disease, allergy, or lactose intolerance since the early 1990s, and are now often attributed to oral ties. Similarly, excessively frequent feeding, excessively broken sleep, and marathon feeding are signs of poor milk transfer, often associated with crying due to poor satiety, but are also still commonly misdiagnosed as signs of GERD, allergy, lactose intolerance, and, most recently, oral ties (Douglas, 2005, 2012, 2013; Douglas & Hill, 2011). These three very common breastfeeding problems are often inappropriately medicalized, still: suboptimal fit and hold, functional lactose overload, and conditioned hyperarousal of the sympathetic nervous system (Douglas & Hill, 2013).

Suboptimal fit and hold leads to suboptimal positional stability, which may result in nipple pain and damage, poor milk transfer, and fussing at the breast. The neurobiological model of infant crying describes the conditioned sympathetic nervous system hyperarousal that occurs if an infant is repeatedly frustrated during breastfeeds by positional instability and poor fit and hold (Douglas & Hill, 2013). Nipple pain is also commonly inappropriately medicalized as due to thrush, or even attributed to functional lactose overload, but (as long as we have excluded unusual medical conditions) is a result of poor fit and hold (Berens et al., 2016). An overly abundant supply may result in both the baby pulling off during the let-down and a functional lactose overload, but won't result in nipple damage if the baby is positionally stable due to optimal fit and hold (Douglas, 2012, 2013).

To further illustrate the scale of the blindspot that we have in our health system concerning clinical breastfeeding support right now, mothers are still widely taught the strategy of shaping the breast with the ipsilateral hand, supporting the infant on the back of the neck, and stimulating a gape before bringing the baby on. Yet this approach has been demonstrated, in Thompson et al.'s (2016) recent large and well-conducted Australian study, to increase the risk of nipple pain fourfold.

The physiological approach to breastfeeding has been a major advance by our clinical breastfeeding support pioneers over the past decade, and is foundational (Schafer & Watson Genna, 2015). However, baby-led breastfeeding is simply not enough for many of our women, who still develop nipple pain and other problems. Multiple well-conducted studies show that currently popular fit and hold strategies, including mammalian methods, do not improve breastfeeding outcomes (De Oliveira et al., 2006; Forster et al., 2004; Henderson & Stamp, 2001; Kronberg & Vaeth, 2009; Kronberg et al., 2012; Labarere et al., 2003; Schafer & Watson Genna, 2015; Wallace et al., 2006).

We have not yet paid enough attention to the complexities of empowering women to fit together with their baby across our gloriously diverse anatomies for pain-free efficient milk transfer. This needs to occur across great diversities of breast shape; breast-tissue elasticity; nipple shape, length, and elasticity; breast-abdominal interface; and infant chin, palate, tongue, lips, and oral connective tissue.

It is not surprising that when clinical approaches are failing, breastfeeding support professionals look at variations of oral connective tissue, and refer for surgical intervention. Yet the breastfeeding problems don't result from tight oral connective tissues but from inadequate health system investment at the frontier of clinical breastfeeding-support skills. The controversy about oral ties in which we find ourselves mired is historically constructed, and no individual's fault; breastfeeding-support professionals are simply doing their absolute best every working day to help mothers, in the context of inadequate health system investment in clinical breastfeeding-support research and training.

To further research in this field, women need a teachable, reproducible, and profoundly empowering approach to fit and hold in breastfeeding. In the hope that it might be helpful for others, we have taken steps to make the Gestalt breastfeeding approach, which we have found so effective in our clinic, widely available (Douglas & Keogh, 2017).

Gestalt breastfeeding builds on the work of our clinical pioneers, to integrate our own clinical experience and new understandings from ultrasound imaging, to empower women as they activate their baby's breastfeeding reflexes and experiment with positional stability and intra-oral breast tissue volume across diverse anatomies. Gestalt breastfeeding also integrates psychological strategies for managing difficult thoughts and feelings.

The digital intra-oral maneuvers and massage interventions of craniosacral therapy, designed to stretch or relax muscles and connective tissue, and teach the tongue new movements, are also based on the same outdated understanding of the biomechanics of infant suck. Unfortunately, a course of craniosacral therapy is an expensive intervention for parents, lacks an evidence-base, and is orally intrusive despite best intentions. Craniosacral therapy, and related techniques, simply cannot compare with healthy effects on postural alignment and functional musculoskeletal health achieved by optimal positional stability, and fit and hold, repeated over and over for many hours each day.

Anything that directs parental financial resource and time investment away from the practice of optimal fit and hold delays the critical repair of the disrupted breastfeeding relationship, and is disempowering for women.

References

Berens, P., Eglash, A., Malloy, M., & Steube, A.M. (2016). Persistent pain with breastfeeding: ABM Clinical Protocol #26. *Breastfeeding Medicine, 11*, 46-56.

De Oliveira, L.D., Giugliani, E.R.J., & do Espirito Santo, L.C. (2006). Effect of intervention to improve breastfeeding technique on the frequency of exclusive breastfeeding and lactation-related problems. *Journal of Human Lactation, 22*, 315-321.

Douglas, P.S. (2005). Excessive crying and gastro-oesophageal reflux disease in infants: misalignment of biology and culture. *Medical Hypotheses, 64*, 887-898.

Douglas, P.S. (2012). Re: Managing infants who cry excessively in the first few months of life. *BMJ*, http://www.bmj.com/content/343/bmj.d7772/rapid-responses.

Douglas, P. (2013). Diagnosing gastro-oesophageal reflux disease or lactose intolerance in babies who cry alot in the first few months overlooks feeding problems. *Journal of Paediatric & Child Health, 49*, e252-256.

Douglas, P., & Hill, P. (2011). Managing infants who cry excessively in the first few months of life. *BMJ, 343*, d7772.

Douglas, P.S., & Hill, P.S. (2013). A neurobiological model for cry-fuss problems in the first three to four months of life. *Medical Hypotheses, 81*, 816-822.

Douglas, P.S., & Keogh, R. (2017, under review). Gestalt breastfeeding: Helping women optimise positional stability and intra-oral breast tissue volume for effective, pain-free milk transfer.

Forster, D., McLachlan, H., Lumley, J., Beanland, C., Waldenstrom, U., & Amir, L. (2004). Two mid-pregnancy interventions to increase the initiation and duration of breastfeeding: a randomized controlled trial. *Birth, 31*, 176-182.

Frymann, V. (1966). Relation of disturbances of craniosacral mechanisms to symptomatology of the newborn: Study of 1,250 infants. *JAOA, 66*, 1059-1075.

Henderson, A., & Stamp, G. (2001). Postpartum positioning and attachment education for increasing breastfeeding: a randomized trial. *Birth, 28*, 236-242.

Herzhaft-Le Roy, J., Xhignesse, M., & Gaboury, I. (2017). Efficacy of an osteopathic treatment coupled with lactation consultations for infants' biomechanical sucking difficulties. *Journal of Human Lactation, 33*(1), 165–172.

Kronborg, H., Maimburg, R. D., & Væth, M. (2012). Antenatal training to improve breast feeding: A randomised trial. *Midwifery, 28*, 784–790.

Kronborg, H., & Væth, M. (2009). How are effective breastfeeding technique and pacifier use related to breastfeeding problems and breastfeeding duration? *Birth, 36*, 34–42.

Labarere, J., Bellin, V., Fourny, M., Gagnaire, J.-C., Francois, P., & Pons J.-C. (2003). Assessment of a structured in-hospital educational intervention addressing breastfeeding: A prospective randomised open trial. *British Journal of Obstetrics and Gynaecology, 110*, 847–852.

Lund, G. C., Edwards, G., Medlin, B., Keller, D., Beck, B., & Carreiro, J. E. (2011). Osteopathic manipulative treatment for the treatment of hospitalized premature infants with nipple feeding dysfunction. *The Journal of the American Osteopathic Association, 111*(1), 44–48.

Maxwell, M. P. R., Fraval, D. O., & Osteo, M. (1998). A pilot study: Osteopathic treatment of infants with a sucking dysfunction. *Journal of the American Academy of Osteopathy, 8*(2), 25–33.

Pizzolorusso, G., Cerritelli, F., D'Orazio, M., Cozzolino, V., Turi, P., Renzetti, C., . . . D'Incecco C. (2013). Osteopathic evaluation of somatic dysfunction and craniosacral strain pattern among preterm and term newborns. *The Journal of the American Osteopathic Association, 113*(6), 462–467.

Schafer, R., & Watson Genna, C. (2015). Physiologic breastfeeding: A contemporary approach to breastfeeding initiation. *Journal of Midwifery & Women's Health, 60*, 546–553.

Thompson, R., Kruske, S., Barclay, L., Linden, K., Gao, Y., & Kildea, S. (2016). Potential predictors of nipple trauma from an in-home breastfeeding programme: A cross-sectional study. *Women and Birth, 29*, 336–344.

Wallace, L. M., Dunn, O. M., Alder, E. M., Inch, S., Hills, R. K., & Law, S. M. (2006). A randomised-controlled trial in England of a postnatal midwifery intervention on breast-feeding duration. *Midwifery, 22*, 262–273.

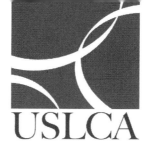

Scope of Practice for IBCLCs and Identifying Tongue-Tie Via Social Media

Keywords: scope of practice; tongue-tie; social media

As we describe in "When Tongue-Ties Were Missed: Mothers' Stories," tongue-tie is often missed, and mothers and babies suffer as a result. Furthermore, many health care providers do not believe that tongue-tie is real. These realities have often left IBCLCs out on the frontiers as possibly the only health care providers in their communities who recognize tongue-tie. In addition, mothers have found experts, and each other, on social media. What is within the Scope of Practice for IBCLCs in these situations? Our panelists describe some of challenges of practicing in the age of social media and when tongue-tie is disregarded. The Scope-of-Practice issues are also described in "IBCLC Scope of Practice for Tongue-Tie Assessment."

What Is Within the Scope of Practice for IBCLCs Regarding Identification of Tongue-Tie?

Catherine Watson Genna

This is a thorny issue. We want to be able to share information with mothers, and our practice guidelines compel us to refer her to health professionals, as appropriate. We need to do this with all due care, and always ensure that the primary health provider of the infant is in the loop, and that the professionals we refer to are not just rubber-stamping our evaluation, but skillfully evaluating the infant themselves. There is evidence that prior diagnosis of a condition affects the judgment of subsequent health care providers.

James Murphy

IBLCE does not permit an IBCLC to make a diagnosis of tongue-tie. I advise IBCLCs to refer a patient with the statement "this infant has demonstrated tongue movement restriction and is having significant breastfeeding difficulty. Please assess for tongue-tie." This tells me that there is a restriction without violating IBLCE rules.

Alison Hazelbaker

Peer supporters, and non-IBCLC lactation educators, and "counselors" have a scope of practice that prevents them from diagnosing. IBCLCs are *expected* to be able to make a tongue-tie lactation diagnosis; it is one of the competencies for lactation consultant practice. Any limits placed on IBCLCs in this regard are based on policies of individual institutions at which an IBCLC may be employed, or on suggestions made in training that IBCLCs do not diagnose. In some countries, IBCLCs are also allowed to perform frenotomy.

The only limit placed on IBCLCs in regard to tongue-tie is lack of skill, and this should be self-imposed. The same is true for any health care professional. If one has not learned how to properly diagnose using an evidence-based screening tool/process, then one should seek out training to learn OR refer to someone who possesses the skill.

Martin Kaplan

The limitation to me would be from the state and national scope of training and education for licensure. Currently, I believe that there is a standard for a licensed IBCLC and RN to diagnose in the scope of their practice. A qualified licensed lactation consultant, RN, NP-IBCLC, PNP-IBCLC, OD, MD, DMD, or DDS has the ability to diagnose for helping support breastfeeding.

Christina Smillie

Well, it's different for me as MD/IBCLC. As best I understand IBLCE's Scope of Practice, IBCLCs are not supposed to "diagnose." Period. But they can certainly describe what they see, which in the case of posterior tongue-tie is really probably the best of what any of us can do: What is the functional mobility? What is the functional capability of this tongue? As far as diagnosis goes, for those of us who are legally expected to diagnose, it's important to remember what we learned early on in training—that you don't just jump to the first diagnosis that comes to mind and then look for proof that the problem is caused by whatever you already think it might be. Especially in complex and confusing situations when we have reason to be uncertain about the likely efficacy of proposed treatment, it is particularly important that we do a careful differential diagnosis: Take a systematic approach to considering what else might it be, consider what are the usual or unusual things that might be confounders, what supports or would refute this assessment, and so forth.

I think one of the reasons lactation consultants may overdiagnose is precisely because diagnosis is considered out of Scope of Practice, and therefore the rules of careful diagnosis aren't taught, aren't on the IBLCE exam. That whole primum non nocere thing is missing. But that doesn't mean these rules of careful diagnosis are arcane or difficult. Really just common sense, logic, and compassion, if you attend to your anatomy and physiology.

Roberta Marinelli and Irene Marchesan

No, there aren't. Any health professional who sees and assesses lingual frenulum must have deep knowledge on lingual frenulum and tongue-tie.

Should Tongue-Tie Be Identified on Social Media?

Alison Hazelbaker

I have two answers to this question. I appreciate the accessibility to information that social media provides. Empowerment based on accurate information delivered in an even-handed, unbiased, and supportive manner can, and should, be championed. Families deserve information that leads to true informed consent. Sites that help a family by supporting them to find properly trained professionals can be applauded.

I deplore those sites that allow non-trained people to diagnose based on description and pictures; these sites not only allow, but somehow encourage bullying, chastisement, shaming, and brow beating. Mothers can support other mothers by *suggesting* screening for tongue-tie by a properly trained professional as a way to rule out tongue-tie as a cause of breastfeeding problems. *No one*, professional *or* lay person, should be making a diagnosis of tongue-tie on a social media site: tongue-tie is a functional problem requiring a functional assessment by a trained professional using an evidence-based screening process.

Any site that pushes mothers into subjecting their babies to treatment without proper diagnosis is potentially causing harm. Because online sites cannot be policed, the owners or moderators of these pages have a duty to run these sites ethically and to hold themselves accountable for the information disseminated. Controlled sites, such as LinkedIn, better ensure ethical behavior. LinkedIn, a site intended for professionals, monitors content posted on all sites and will block content that does not meet ethical standards.

Carmela Baeza

Many mothers know more about breastfeeding that health care providers. I often receive dyads who have been referred to me by mothers, who perhaps had breastfeeding problems because of tongue-tie themselves and can therefore identify the problem. Or simply, they have read good, accurate information. So I believe mothers can certainly help each other this way.

There is a dark side, however. Wrong diagnosis might be given, which can on the one side create unnecessary worry, and on the other hand increase the risk of unnecessary interventions or delay correct diagnosis of other difficulties. I would ask mothers on social media sites to refer other mothers to certified lactation consultants.

Catherine Watson Genna

Humans seem to pass through a stage where we think we know everything before learning that we really know very little. It is uncomfortable to live with ambiguity. I think these forums help mothers who were traumatized by difficult breastfeeding because of undiagnosed tongue-tie to attempt to help other people (part of the human drive to "redeem" hard experiences). They do create a lot of concern and demand for treatment before children have ever been evaluated by a professional. I am being contacted by more and more of these mothers who went straight to a practitioner to have the frenulum divided, without any improvement in breastfeeding. It's really hard to determine then if there was ever really a tongue-tie, or if there were breastfeeding management or other difficulties.

James Murphy

Until primary care physicians step up to the plate, and properly and consistently assess each newborn infant for a tongue-tie, and make an appropriate referral, moms have to stick together and help each other. I have patients referred to my office rather often from another mother on one of the social-media platforms. They are usually correct in their assessment. IBLCE has no rules on moms making such a diagnosis.

Christina Smillie

Mothers want to do the best for their babies, and oxytocin just makes everything around both babies and feeding so emotionally laden. A look at these sites can break your heart. A lesson I hope in humility for us all. The harm that can be done when a single diagnosis has been so promoted by our profession that mothers are willing to subject their infants to a somewhat noxious procedure they know little about, because they care so much for their babies.

We are the ones who need to take heed of how our words echo and reverberate into chambers far beyond our own. Another *Primum non nocere.*

Roberta Martinelli and Irene Marchesan

Sharing experiences is always healthy. Mothers can provide information for other mothers to be aware of possible tongue-tie. When mothers are in doubt whether the lingual frenulum of the baby is altered or not, a breastfeeding and frenulum specialist must be asked about revision.

Martin Kaplan

The sites available for the public to research are wonderful. When a mother presents to me with her own diagnosis, I always ask where she learned about the tongue-tie. I use this as a starting point to compliment her on her research. Then we go through the intake forms, and check-off lists that I use in my office to start a conversation. I must add that I would hope the mother would have seen an IBCLC, CLC, MD, or DO, or NP etc. first, as there certainly could be other factors that affect lack of successful breastfeeding as was previously mentioned.

Unfortunately, there is a distrust of the medical and dental profession and mothers are relying on their own personal experience to assist other mothers. Many will take the social media contact advice, and make a decision whether to follow up with treatment or not.

The ways we combat these negatives is by supporting the mothers and acknowledge their effort to learn and be proactive. Then, we must earn their confidence and guide them through the diagnosis and potential treatments for surgery, body work, or more lactation guidance.

Pamela Douglas

Social media is a powerful and overwhelmingly positive tool for mothers supporting mothers. However, women are reliant on the information that health professionals offer them. Therefore, I don't like to blame mothers on social media who are simply acting on the inaccurate information given to them by health professionals, either in consultations, or on health professional websites and blogs.

Instead, I do think the breastfeeding community needs to take a stand against the destructive "groupthink" that has taken hold amongst some breastfeeding support professionals.

Groupthink is a well-known psychological phenomenon that occurs when the desire to belong within a group of people results in dysfunctional decision-making. Groupthink requires active suppression of dissenting viewpoints, and in health care, can result in what has been called "the medical-miracles delusion" (Braithwaite, 2014). When groupthink is active, those who dissent intellectually may find themselves excluded, denigrated, or their incomes put at risk, through the compilation of online preferred provider lists, through blogs and private Facebook posts questioning their competence, experience, or professionalism, and through various other mechanisms.

It grieves me to hear of personal and professional damage being done to courageous individuals who dare to speak out against yet another trend to unnecessary medicalization in the care of breastfeeding mothers and their babies. It is such a vulnerable time of life. Mothers and babies need their health professionals to be freely engaged in the most robust and inclusive intellectual debates possible!

Reference

Braithwaite, J. (2014). The medical miracles delusion. *The Royal Society of Medicine*, 107, 92-93.

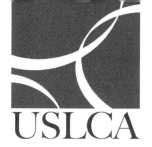

IBCLC Scope of Practice for Tongue-Tie Assessment

Elizabeth Brooks, JD, IBCLC, FILCA

Keywords: scope of practice; tongue-tie; ankyloglossia; IBLCE; IBCLC; practice-guiding document; professionalism

There is vigorous debate in the research, academic, public health, and clinical communities serving families with infants about the impact of infant ankyloglossia ("tongue-tie") on effective breastfeeding and lactation. Will a tethered tongue (and perhaps even tethered lips and cheeks) negatively impact lactation and result in suboptimal breastfeeding and early weaning? What options can we offer families who seek relief from nipple pain, low-weight gain, and distressed babies? These are legitimate questions, but a more elementary examination is whether it is within the scope of practice for the IBCLC to assess the infant's oral cavity, observe a feed-at-breast, and share concerns with the primary health care provider. This article reviews the practice-guiding documents relevant to ethical and clinical care by an IBCLC and highlights the authority that allows the IBCLC to offer evidence-based information and support, including a comprehensive feeding assessment, for the baby suspected of tongue-tie.

Ankyloglossia ("Tongue-Tie"), Generally

To state the obvious, we know that infants and children who are feeding at breast use their mouths to do so, and we know the tongue plays an important role in allowing for effective latch and suckling. Indeed, amongst the numerous elements contained in the certification examination conducted by the International Board of Lactation Consultant Examiners® (IBLCE®) to award the International Board Certified Lactation Consultant® (IBCLC®) credential are knowledge of "infant anatomy and anatomical/oral challenges" and "ankyloglossia" (IBLCE, 2014, at I.A.3. and III.A.2). The IBCLC should be able to know how to spot tongue-tie, to tell families how this impacts lactation, and be able to educate them about care options they can explore with the primary health care provider (HCP) for the child.

Scope of Practice, Generally

A "scope of practice" (SOP) describes everything a practitioner, in any health care profession, is entitled to do, as part of the clinical and instructional interaction with patients/clients. It might be a document enforced (via a disciplinary process) by a governmental entity that issues a license, required to be held by all practitioners, if they plan to see clients/patients. It might be something enforced by the professional association for that practitioner group.

The right to issue a license, define a scope of practice, and have a disciplinary process (to remove illegitimate or ill-performing practitioners) all spring from the legal authority allowing regulations to protect the public's health, safety, and welfare. The notion is: If health care providers (HCPs) are going to "hang out a shingle," and start charging money to see families, and discuss clinical care plans, or perform rudimentary or even invasive procedures, we members of the public want assurance that HCPs have met minimal standards of education and training.

We want to feel that the folks providing care know what they are doing, and are able to do it well. And if they are terrible clinicians, or they engage in unprofessional behaviors, despite excellent clinical skill, we want a means to file a complaint about them, with their right to practice – the license – held in the balance. All of this is in addition to whatever lawsuits we may legitimately bring, under various tort theories (Brooks, 2013).

Many of those with the IBCLC credential have a license *in addition to* the IBCLC certification they received from IBLCE. The scope of practice for those other licenses (i.e., registered nurse, physician, midwife, neonatal nurse practitioner, dentist, speech/language therapist, chiropractor, occupational therapist, physical therapist, etc.) may well encompass the ability to assess infant oral structures and feeding capabilities, to *diagnose* certain conditions, and even to perform clinical invasive procedures to correct tongue-tie. Thus, some IBCLCs may indeed be seeing, assessing, diagnosing, and correcting a tongue-tie. But their authority to do so springs from the scope of practice associated with the other license.

For purposes of this article, we will not discuss those clinicians who are IBCLC *in addition to* something else. We will assume they are excellently practicing, and excellently serving families with tongue-tie, because it is within their various licenses and scopes of practice to do so. Instead, we will focus on the legitimate range of assessment and care about tongue-tie that IBCLCs are able to offer when they have the stand-alone IBCLC credential as their sole certification to provide skilled breastfeeding and human lactation care.

Scope of Practice for the IBCLC

The IBCLC has three major, **mandatory practice-guiding documents**, all enforced by the International Board of Lactation Consultant Examiners.

1. IBLCE *Code of Professional Conduct for IBCLCs* ("IBLCE CPC") (IBLCE, 2015a), which requires the IBCLC at Principle 8 to comply with the IBLCE *Disciplinary Procedures for the Code of Professional Conduct for IBCLCs for the International Board of Lactation Consultant Examiners (IBLCE)* (IBLCE, 2016)

2. IBLCE *Scope of Practice for International Board Certified Lactation Consultant (IBCLC) Certificants* ("IBLCE SOP") (IBLCE, 2012a)

3. IBLCE *Clinical Competencies for the Practice of International Board Certified Lactation Consultants (IBCLCs)* ("IBLCE CC") (IBLCE, 2012b).

These three documents are interdependent: The IBLCE Clinical Competencies (CC) describes in detail the clinical skills that "encompass the responsibilities/activities that are part of the IBCLC's practice" (IBLCE, 2012b, p. 1), and further requires IBCLCs to conduct themselves "in a professional manner" by "practicing within the framework defined by the IBLCE CPC, the IBLCE SOP and the IBLCE CC" (ibid.).

There are also **voluntary practice-guiding documents** relevant to an IBCLC's care for a family where tongue-tie is problematic. They are:

1. Two advisory opinions of IBLCE, on frenulotomy, and social media presence of the IBCLC (IBLCE, 2013; IBLCE, 2015b)

2. ILCA Standards of Practice for International Board Certified Lactation Consultants ("ILCA Standards") (ILCA, 2013)

IBLCE Clinical Competencies (CC)

Several sections of the IBLCE CC describe the IBCLC's ability to make a skilled assessment for something like suspected tongue-tie, in order to share information with the family and their primary healthcare provider. Relevant elements:

1. The IBCLC has the duty to provide competent services for mothers and families and will perform a comprehensive maternal, child and feeding assessment related to lactation, such as: [A]ssess oral anatomy and normal neurological responses and reflexes ... identify correct latch/attachment ... assess effective milk transfer ... assess for adequate milk intake of the child

   ... provide evidence-based information to assist the mother to make informed decisions regarding breastfeeding intake ... provide information and strategies to prevent and resolve painful, damaged nipples ... facilitate breastfeeding for the medically fragile and physically compromised child

   ... provide anticipatory guidance to reduce potential risks to the breastfeeding mother or her child ... assess and provide strategies to initiate and continue breastfeeding when challenging situations exist/occur ... critique and evaluate indications, contraindication and use of techniques, appliances and devices which support breastfeeding ... provide evidence-informed information to the mother regarding the use of techniques and devices

   ... provide evidence-informed information regarding complementary therapies during lactation and their impact on a mother's milk production and the effect on her child ... provide support and encouragement to enable mothers to successfully meet their breastfeeding goals ... support the mother to make evidence-informed decisions for her child and herself.

2. The IBCLC has the duty to act with reasonable diligence and will: [A]ssist families with decisions regarding feeding their children by providing evidence-informed information that is free of any conflicts of interest ... make appropriate referrals to other health care providers and community support resources in a timely manner depending on the urgency of the situation ... work collaboratively with the health care team to provide coordinated services to families (IBLCE CC, 2012b, pp.2-4).

IBLCE Scope of Practice (SOP)

The language of the IBLCE is nearly identical to that of the IBLCE CC. It is affirmational: it describes what an IBCLC **can** do; it is silent about prohibited activities. Thus, IBCLCs have "demonstrated specialized knowledge and clinical expertise in breastfeeding and human lactation," and, the IBLCE SOP "encompasses activities for which IBCLC certificants are educated and in which they are authorized to engage" (IBLCE SOP, 2012a, p 1). It elaborates practice skills for assessing suspected tongue-tie, sharing evidence-based information and support with the family, and alerting the primary HCP about this clinical concern:

IBCLC certificants have the duty to provide competent services for mothers and families by: [P]erforming comprehensive maternal, child and feeding assessments related to lactation ... providing evidence-based information regarding complementary therapies during lactation and their impact on a mother's milk product and the effect on her child ... providing support and encouragement to enable mothers to successfully meet their breastfeeding goals.

IBCLC certificants have the duty to act with reasonable diligence by: [A]ssisting families with decisions regarding the feeding of children by providing information that is evidence-based and free of any conflicts of interest ... making appropriate referrals to other health care providers and community support resources when necessary ... working collaboratively and interdependently with other members of the health care team (IBLCE SOP, 2012a, paras. 5 & 8).

IBLCE Code for Professional Conduct (CPC)

The IBLCE CPC, the mandatory ethical code for IBCLC professional behaviors, "[p]rovides IBCLCs with a framework for carrying out their essential duties [and] serves as a basis for decision regarding alleged misconduct" (IBLCE CPC, 2015a, p 1). Within it, several principles underscore the professional assessment and information-sharing parameters described in the IBLCE CC and IBLCE SOP for competent evaluation of tongue-tie, and indeed, *require* that every IBCLC shall:

1.1 Fulfill professional commitment by working with mothers to meet their breastfeeding goals

1.3 supply sufficient and accurate information to enable clients to make informed decisions

2.1 Operate within the limits of the scope of practice

2.2 Collaborate with other members of the health care team to provide united and comprehensive care

4.1 Receive a client's consent, before initiate a consultation, to share clinical information with other members of the client's health care team.

7.1 Operate within the framework defined by the CPC. (IBLCE CPC, 2015a, pp. 1-3).

IBLCE Advisory Opinions

IBLCE has issued only two Advisory Opinions in its history, and both are relevant to an examination of an IBCLC's scope of practice for tongue-tie assessment. The first, the *IBLCE Advisory Opinion – Frenulotomy* ("IBLCE Advisory 1") (IBLCE, 2013) addresses the situation of IBCLCs actually performing frenulotomies to remedy tongue-tie. It recognizes that "frenulotomy is not expressly covered in the IBLCE SOP," and is not an authorized procedure for IBCLCs "unless they are separately licensed or authorized to perform frenulotomies" in their geopolitical region (IBLCE Advisory 1, 2013, p. 1).

This echoes our conclusions, above, that IBCLCs who have *other* licenses may have broader clinical authority than the stand-alone IBCLC, including ability to perform tongue-tie related corrections. But the IBCLC certification on its own does not confer the training and expertise to perform frenulotomies (IBLCE, 2013). Nonetheless, IBCLC certification certainly confers through the IBLCE CPC, SOP and CC broad powers to *assess* for tongue-tie, offer *evidence-based information and support* to the family to understand how this will impact their infant feeding goals, and *share clinical concerns* with the primary health care providers.

IBLCE Advisory Opinion: Professionalism in the Social Media Age ("IBLCE Advisory 2") (IBLCE, 2015b) is meant to be read together with the IBLCE CPC and IBCLE SOP. It cautions the IBCLC about using electronic forms of communication and Internet-based social media to perform consultations, because of "inherent difficulties of not being able to perform an examination of the breast and infant's oral anatomy and the inability to observe the latch and feeding in person" (IBLCE Advisory 2, 2015b, p. 2). The undeniable conclusion is that the IBCLC *does* have the skill and ability, per the IBLCE CPC and IBLCE SOP, to perform a thorough oral assessment (which would uncover oral tethers and tongue-tie) precisely because IBLCE wants this to be happening in person, and not over the Internet.

Update from IBLCE

Just as *Clinical Lactation* was about to go to press for this issue, the International Board of Lactation Consultant Examiners issued *Advisory Opinion: Assessment, Diagnosis, and Referral** (the third in their history) (AO 3), addressing the appropriate scope of practice for an IBCLC whose patient/client has suspected tongue-tie. It succinctly offers authority for the very advice underpinning this article's analysis: Excellent IBCLC care is about offering evidence-based information and support.

The IBCLC does not "practice medicine," nor offer a "medical diagnosis" or "treatment" (as AO 3 defines these terms) **unless** the IBCLC has **another** license or certification providing scope of practice/authority to do so. Of interest is the Addendum to AO 3, offering sample scripts an IBCLC may use when discussing tongue-tie, thrush, mastitis, and use of milk-boosting herbs.

The moral of the story for the IBCLC is: offer evidence-based information and support, so the family can make an informed decision about the parent's and the baby's health care, after discussion with the primary health care provider. The full text of AO 3 may be downloaded on their website (http://iblce.org/wp-content/uploads/2013/08/advisory-opinion-assessment-diagnosis-referral-english.pdf).

ILCA Standards

The International Lactation Consultant Association issues an important voluntary practice-guiding document for IBCLCs. IBCLCs and others who support the organization may choose to become members of this international professional association. Regardless of membership status, any IBCLC may follow the standards described in the document. Unlike the IBLCE CPC, IBLCE SOP, and IBLCE CC, there is no disciplinary process to enforce these guidelines at ILCA. They are best practices, intended to be voluntarily met by excellently practicing IBCLCs. The ILCA Standards are "a set of guidelines that define the tasks and skills the IBCLCs should be able to perform in the course of fulfilling the duties of the profession" (ILCA standards, 2013, p 1). To wit, relevant portions:

> [In] all interactions with clients/patients, families and other health care professionals, the IBCLC should adhere to [the ILCA Standards, IBLCE CPC, IBLCE SOP, IBLCE CC] ...

> 1.4 Act as an advocate for breastfeeding women, infants, and children

> 1.5 Assist the mother in maintaining a breastfeeding relationship with her child ...

> [Focus] on providing clinical lactation care and management. This is best accomplished by promoting optimal health through collaboration and problem-solving with the patient/client and other members of the health care team. The role of the IBCLC includes assessment, planning, intervention, and evaluation in a variety of situations;

anticipatory guidance and prevention of problems; communication and collaboration with other health care professionals ...

Systematically collect objective and subjective information

3.1.3. Discuss all assessment information with the mother and documents as appropriate

3.2.1. Analyze assessment information to identify issues and/ or problems

3.2.2. Develop a plan of care based on identified issues

3.2.3. Arrange or refer for follow-up evaluation where indicated ...

3.3.5. Facilitate referral to other health care professional, community services and support groups as needed ...

3.3.7 Document and communicate to health care providers [a] ssessment information, suggested interventions, instructions provided, evaluations of outcomes, modifications of the plan of care, and follow-up strategies ...

4.1 Educate parents and families to encourage informed decisions about infant and child feeding...

4.3 Provide anticipatory guidance (teaching) to promote optimal breastfeeding practices and minimize the potential for problems or complications

4.5 Share current, evidence-based information and clinical skills in collaboration with other health care providers (ILCA Standards, 2013, pp. 1-4).

Can an IBCLC Diagnose Tongue-Tie?

Under the IBLCE SOP, the answer is: No. Recall the IBLCE SOP describes affirmational skills that the IBCLC is able to engage in; it is not a list of prohibited activities. A review of the all of the mandatory practice-guiding documents reveals that IBCLCS are—repeatedly—given authority to *assess and inform*. But there is NO mention of the right/ability to *diagnose* a medical condition. Its absence from the practice-guiding documents means IBCLCs are not vested with the ability to *diagnose* tongue-tie.

But any-and-everything-else is right in the IBCLC bailiwick: Show the family how and why the oral examination is being done; inform them about what is being observed and how this fits with (and can explain) the overall lactation problems (pain, injury, low milk supply, long and ineffectual feeds, slow weight gain); explain that an actual diagnosis is made by the child's primary health care provider, but ineffective breastfeeding history is an important element to consider; describe treatment options the family might discuss with the primary health care provider (including frenulotomy and appropriate wound care after such a procedure); devise a lactation care plan to protect milk supply and feed the baby while all care options are considered for the tongue-tie ... including the family's decision not to have it revised.

Conclusion

What does all of this seeming legalese mean for the practitioner?

1. An IBCLC (who practices under that stand-alone credential, alone) is required to have expert clinical knowledge about ankyloglossia just to pass the certification exam.

2. In providing clinical care to families, in a manner that protects the public's health, safety, and welfare, an IBCLC is able to *assess* for tongue-tie, offer *evidence-based information*

and support to the family to understand how this will impact their infant-feeding goals, and *share clinical concerns* with the primary HCPs.

3. The primary health care provider diagnoses tongue tie. A health care provider (a dentist, doctor, neonatal nurse practitioner, midwife, oral surgeon), who is trained in providing frenulotomies or tongue-tie revisions can perform such procedures. The IBCLC practicing solely on the stand-alone certification cannot diagnose, and cannot perform corrective procedures.

4. Tongue-tie assessment is best done hands-on, and face-to-face, because in-person consultations allow for effective evaluation of breastfeeding and human lactation. This may involve visual and digital examination of the baby's oral cavity, using sensible universal precautions.

5. A critical role the IBCLC plays is to educate the family, and health care practitioner colleagues, about the role of the tongue in effective breastfeeding, and how oral restriction can have a negative impact on feeding which result in the family not meeting its infant feeding goals.

References

Brooks, E. (2013). *Legal and ethical issues for the IBCLC*. Burlington, MA: Jones & Bartlett.

International Board of Lactation Consultant Examiners. (2012a, September 15). *Scope of practice for international board certified lactation consultant (IBCLC) certificants*. Retrieved February 21, 2017, from International Board of Lactation Consultant Examiners website: http://iblce.org/wp-content/uploads/2013/08/scope-of-practice.pdf

International Board of Lactation Consultant Examiners. (2012b, September 15). *Clinical competencies for the practice of international board certified lactation consultants (IBCLCs)*. Retrieved February 21, 2017, from International Board of Lactation Consultant Examiners website: http://iblce.org/wp-content/uploads/2013/08/clinical-competencies.pdf

International Board of Lactation Consultant Examiners. (2013, February). *International board of lactation consultant examiners (IBLCE): Advisory opinion*

- *frenulotomy*. Retrieved February 24, 2017, from International Board of Lactation Consultant Examiners website: http://iblce.org/wp-content/uploads/2013/08/advisory-opinion-frenulotomy-english.pdf

International Board of Lactation Consultant Examiners. (2014). *International board of lactation consultant examiners (IBCLE) international board certified lactation consultant (IBCLC) detailed content outline [effective January 2016]*. Retrieved February 23, 2017, from International Board of Lactation Consultant Examiners website: http://iblce.org/wp-content/uploads/2013/08/IBCLC-Detailed-Content-Outline-for-2016-for-Publication.pdf

International Board of Lactation Consultant Examiners. (2015a, September). *Code of professional conduct for IBCLCs*. Retrieved February 21, 2017, from International Board of Lactation Consultant Examiners website: http://iblce.org/wp-content/uploads/2013/08/Code-of-professional-conduct.pdf

International Board of Lactation Consultant Examiners. (2015b, September). *Advisory opinion: Professionalism in the social media age*. Retrieved February 24, 2017, from International Board of Lactation Consultant Examiners website: http://iblce.org/wp-content/uploads/2016/01/Advisory-Opinion-Social-Media-Professionalism.pdf

International Board of Lactation Consultant Examiners. (2016, November 3). *Disciplinary procedures for the code of professional conduct for IBCLCs for the international board of lactation consultant examiners (IBLCE)*. Retrieved February 23, 2017, from International Board of Lactation Consultant Examiners website: http://iblce.org/wp-content/uploads/2013/08/disciplinary-procedures-2.pdf

International Board of Lactation Consultant Examiners. (2017, March 22). *Advisory opinion: Assessment, diagnosis, and referral*. Retrieved from International Board of Lactation Consultant Examiners website: http://iblce.org/wp-content/uploads/2013/08/advisory-opinion-assessment-diagnosis-referral-english.pdf

International Lactation Consultant Association. (2013, December). *Standards of practice for international board certified lactation consultants*. Retrieved February 21, 2017, from International Lactation Consultant Association website: https://goo.gl/D3QnZ6

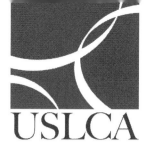

USLCA

When Tongue-Ties Were Missed: Mothers' Stories

Keywords: breastfeeding problems; sore nipples; tongue-tie

When we asked for mothers to tell us their stories of tongue-tie, responses flooded in. A theme in many of these stories is health care providers not listening when mothers said they were in pain. The mothers' related stories of painful nipples, babies breastfeeding "all the time," and failure to thrive because of low milk production. Mothers' voices were not heard because health-care providers minimized their concerns. Most of these mothers persisted with breastfeeding despite the problems. Eventually, the tongue-ties were correctly identified and revised, and the difficulties resolved. Other mothers were not able to continue breastfeeding. A smaller percentage of mothers described revisions that had harmful effects on their babies and that did not fix the breastfeeding problems.

Amy

Amy's daughter is 4 months. Feeding is going well now, but she struggled for 4 to 6 weeks with sore nipples that made her cry with pain and frustration. Health care providers did not listen to her concerns. She felt like a failure.

> ... I had a real feeling that something wasn't right with my daughter too, and tried to get our lactation consultants and doctor to diagnose tongue-tie, but they were inexplicably not prepared to do so, insisting that they weren't qualified to.
>
> After weeks of using a nipple shield to protect my incredibly sore nipples ... I finally insisted that we were referred to an ENT specialist. I am no doctor, but I just knew something wasn't right. Finally, my doctor relented and referred us, and lo and behold, the ENT specialist immediately confirmed my suspicions, diagnosed her with tongue-tie, and snipped it then and there. It was upsetting, but such a relief to have my suspicions validated. It didn't make a huge difference straight away, but over the weeks it's helped so much.

Her sister, living in the UK, had a similar experience and struggled for a month. Once the tongue-tie addressed, "it was a life changer."

Jamie

Jamie made a video of her experience with a baby with tongue-tie. You can see her story here.

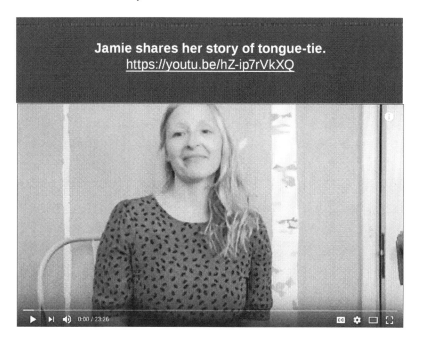

Jamie shares her story of tongue-tie.
https://youtu.be/hZ-ip7rVkXQ

Angela

A hospital lactation consultant told Angela that her late preterm baby was a "lazy nurser," and she never checked for a tie. Although her baby gained well, they struggled with breastfeeding for 3 and a half months.

> I met with a lactation consultant, and they verified he had a tongue- and lip-tie. The next week, we had an appointment with a pediatric dentist to have it revised via laser. All went well, and we got through the aftercare, but it was difficult for all of us. The spitting up and excessive gas cleared up in the weeks post-revision. He also got more efficient at nursing

111

because it was taking him much less time/feed. He's 15 months now and still breastfeeding, along with eating everything we put in front of him! Overall, I'm very happy with how our revision turned out and I'm glad we did it. I wish we would have known sooner.

Rebecca

Rebecca was adamant about breastfeeding until her son naturally weaned, even as she struggled with pain and feeding nearly every hour.

> Our maternal-child nurse, who is also a lactation consultant, basically told me I was doing it all wrong! I had parents whose babies were stars with solids ... telling me to give him carrot sticks, bread sticks and all sorts of crazy things! He just didn't deal with it well at all! He wasn't gaining weight like he should, and my maternal-child health nurse, and my family began blaming it on me breastfeeding him too often. I was told if I cut back on feeds he would eat more. I didn't listen to this advice as I wasn't comfortable with it.

The problems continued. Her baby started having speech and language problems, as well as ongoing issues with solid food.

> At 14 months, he was having speech problems and trouble swallowing food. The speech pathologist told her to cut the breastfeeds and offer more food.

She finally saw her osteopath, who diagnosed a very tight posterior tie and lip-tie, and referred the baby for laser correction.

> This was probably the most difficult moment of my life. ... However, it was the best decision I have made! It took

a little while, but within a few months he was talking more, finally saying dad, and swallowing his food! He even started sleeping longer stretches!

She described her second baby as "a star feeder from the beginning," but "... even in hospital I could see she had a shallow latch, a lip-tie, a very high palate, she was clicking on the breast, and taking in more air than anything else." The baby was referred to have a tongue- and lip-tie correction.

> ... we had a fortnight of horrendous nights due to stretches, but it all calmed down after that. ... my tight uncomfortable baby was now a loose comfortable bub! She was latching much better, and now at 5 months old is an old pro on the breast! It could be coincidence, but she also sleeps through most nights.

Bree

Bree found the answer to her issues via Facebook. Her baby was gaining well, but she had cracked and bleeding nipples, which she said she had been "prepared to deal with." Her son's posterior tongue- and upper lip-tie were released when her baby was 5 months old. She thought her baby had reflux, but someone suggested that she see a lactation consultant first, before he started on medication, who suspected a tongue-tie and made a referral.

> When I was in the hospital after delivering, I kept telling the nurses it hurts and it's not right. He was never flanging his lips. He was not getting a good seal. They just kept saying keep trying it will come. Then they would scurry off somewhere else. I felt defeated and incompetent. I finally went home out of sheer frustration. Hoping my comfy house would give me relief.

Things did get better for her after the release. Less pain and her baby stopped spitting up so much.

Chrissy

Chrissy had Placenta Previa and had her daughter via planned cesarean. Her baby was taken away for the first hour. They tried breastfeeding after that, but her daughter didn't latch right away and breastfed sporadically while in the hospital. The lactation consultant said her latch looked good, but that she needed to do more skin to skin, which she did. Chrissy and her baby were discharged after 48 hours.

Their first night home was "horrible." Her baby screamed, and when she would finally latch, it was excruciating. Her husband bought a pump the next morning as soon as the store opened, and Chrissy was able to pump 4 ounces of breast milk.

> The public health nurse came to visit us that day and was impressed with my milk output from pumping, and told us the latch looked great, but sometimes nursing hurts for the first little while.

All the health care providers she saw minimized or ignored her painful breastfeeding for the next 3 ½ weeks. She also received some outdated advice.

> The first 10 to 25 seconds after a latch took my breath away, and made my toes curl with a pain I had never before experienced. The rest of a nursing session was painful enough that when my husband was home he would hold my hand and stroke my hair while I nursed our daughter and cried.

> ... I saw two more lactation consultants, one of whom told me I could try "toughening up" my nipples by

"rubbing them with a washcloth," and two doctors as well. We were diagnosed with thrush, though neither Gentian Violet nor Nystatin did anything to lessen the symptoms.

Other mothers were the ones who told Chrissy to look into possible lip- or tongue-ties.

> ... I asked both lactation consultants and both doctors about this. All four of them told me that she had no ties, and her latch looked good. None of them seemed to believe how much pain nursing caused me, and formula was suggested multiple times.

> ... By this point I was becoming desperate, but I KNEW that nursing was NOT supposed to be like this. There was absolutely NO possible way I could continue nursing under those conditions, and I was days away from giving up and buying formula.

She finally contacted a lactation consultant over video chat, who diagnosed tongue- and lip-tie, as well as vasospasm of the nipples. The lactation consultant referred her to a pediatric dentist closer to her home, who confirmed by posterior tongue- and lip-tie.

> We opted to do a laser revision that day, and the difference in the width of my daughter's mouth in the before and after photos is astonishing. I nursed her mere minutes after the revision, and it was painless for me for the first time ever. She nursed for about 15 minutes, and then unlatched and looked around happily. The difference was incredible. We did stretches 5 times per day for six weeks to prevent the ties from reattaching, and my nipples gradually healed.

She would have weaned if she had not, finally, gotten the correct diagnosis.

> I am 100% certain that I would have stopped nursing within a couple of days if we had never spoken with the IBCLC who diagnosed the ties. Instead, my daughter is 17 months and still nursing happily; we are just beginning to think about the weaning process now.

Emma

Emma's second child was having trouble breastfeeding right from the start. She could never latch and would slide right off the nipple. She would scream and vomit copiously. Emma had a good milk supply, with a forceful letdown, so her baby "was essentially force fed."

> ... Because I had had the positive breastfeeding experience with my son I knew within the first 24 hours after her birth it wasn't right. I told the midwives, asked to see the hospital LC and everyone told me it looked fine. ... She was gaining weight and I wasn't experiencing any pain so every health professional I spoke to told me there was no problem. Expect there was.

Her baby never slept, and would vomit so much that she "filled her bassinet." Emma was terrified, so she wasn't sleeping either. She finally found a lactation consultant who finally stuck her fingers in her baby's mouth, and diagnosed an upper lip-tie and posterior tongue-tie.

> ... A few days later we had the ties revised and immediately afterwards my daughter's latch was dramatically improved. It still took a few weeks for it to

become 100%, but there was a significant improvement for my daughter straight away. She stopped vomiting. Slept better. Fed for longer stretches and was just generally happier.

Because she was an experienced mother, she kept looking for answers. She, too, would have weaned. Emma correctly recognizes that this was a problem with the health care system, not the mothers.

> ... If I hadn't of had the experience with my first, I wouldn't have known to continue arguing that there was something wrong with my daughter's latch. I would have listened to the health processionals, and assumed that was what breastfeeding was like. I would have given up on breastfeeding, assuming I was just another one of those women who "failed to breastfeed." But in actual fact, I wouldn't have failed at breastfeeding. The health care system would have failed *me* to provide me with the proper support and treatment to establish and maintain breastfeeding. It needs to change.

Erin K.

Erin is a nurse practitioner, who struggled with breastfeeding in the hospital. She left with "with my pockets stuffed with formula." She continued to have a difficult time at home, and finally saw a lactation consultant, who helped her a lot. She was able to breastfeed her first baby for 16 months.

Because she had one good breastfeeding experience, she knew something wasn't right with her second baby, who couldn't latch. It was her doula who first spotted the tongue-tie. She was referred to a pediatric dentist, but had to wait 6 weeks for an appointment. Breastfeeding was "torturous" during that time, and her nipples developed ulcers.

> The day my daughter saw the oral surgeon, he performed a laser procedure of both the tongue- and lip-ties. Roughly 10 minutes after the procedure, had me breastfeed her. It was like night and day. Although tender from the damage that had already been done, I knew that something had changed and it felt "right." I've had no issues since. My daughter is now 17.5 months and continues to breastfeed.

She probably would have weaned had she not gotten help.

> I would like to think I would have persevered to 6 months despite the pain, etc. had I not had the procedure, but perhaps that's not realistic. I certainly wouldn't have made it as far as we have.

Erin R.

Erin R.'s breastfeeding struggles contributed to her postpartum depression. She and her baby were both miserable, and her baby was losing weight.

> He couldn't stay latched, and we spend nearly all feeds crying. My little boy screaming in frustration of not being able to latch and stay on, and myself as I couldn't feed my baby.

She was ready to quite when her health visitor correctly diagnosed a tongue-tie.

> The tongue-tie was snipped and reviewed for the following week. At this review, his tie was snipped again. Our breastfeeding journey is now nearly 9 months in.

I'm grateful for the service provided when finally have tongue-tie snipped, but very disappointed no one checked before then especially with all the difficulties I was having. I really feel it was a major part in my PND [postnatal depression]!

Heather

Heather started pumping exclusively for her twins, as she was told they were "too weak to latch." When they were released from the hospital, she would put them to breast, but they were slow feeders, and it was painful for her. The pediatrician blamed the problems on their prematurity, and urged her to keep pumping. By 3 months, she'd had mastitis twice, weekly clogged milk ducts, and sore, cracked, and bleeding nipples. Her supply dropped, and she became depressed. The babies were on medication for GERD. A friend thought her babies might be tongue-tied.

> Our ped again said it was just because they were premature. My supply began dropping as I continued to struggle not knowing where else to turn, and my postpartum depression grew with each bad latch. I felt horrible for wanting to quit, thought it just must be something wrong with me, that I wasn't strong enough.

A La Leche League leader referred her to another doctor when she "couldn't take it anymore." The doctor corrected both a tongue- and lip-tie.

> ... and I never experienced pain again. My supply, unfortunately, had decreased so much at that point that I wasn't able to exclusively breastfeed.

She was able to partially breastfeed for about 13 months, and now helps other mothers.

We never would have made it that far without having the ties corrected. My girls are now happy and healthy 5-year-olds, and I spend my days as a certified postpartum doula to help moms avoid experiences like mine. I hope to one day become a certified lactation counselor, and I am actually the receptionist in a private practice that helps moms with tongue-ties. I am very passionate about turning my bad experience into good outcomes for new moms.

Jacqueline

Jacqueline had three babies who were all tongue-tied to varying degrees. With her first baby, the pediatrician noticed a classic tongue-tie right away,

> ... but told me there was nothing to do about it as long as he was gaining weight okay. By 3 days of life, my baby had regained his birth weight, my milk was in, and my nipples were cracked, bleeding, scabbed, and I was in excruciating pain with every single latch. I requested a referral to have my son's tie evaluated, but our pediatrician denied my request due to my son's more-than- adequate weight gain, and let me know if it caused speech problems it would be addressed at that time.

Her insurance didn't cover an IBCLC. She endured "extreme pain" with every feeding for 6 weeks. She was a CLC, and did what she could to minimize the pain.

> ...There were times I wanted to throw my baby off of my breast, and I cried at the thought him latching. I felt like a robot. I had no feelings of love for him, our bonding was beyond impaired. Just writing this

brings me to tears because he and I were robbed of such a crucial time in our relationship, and we were failed by those whose job it was to help us. We went on to breastfeed for 18 months.

She still feels trauma symptoms from that time, and her son had continuous health problems because his tongue-tie was not addressed.

Jaqueline's second baby was born 5 weeks before she sat for her IBCLC exam. She didn't see an anterior tie, but had pain, nipples that were white after feedings, and a pinched line on her nipples. Her baby was a noisy nurser, and burped loudly.

My hospital IBCLC told me that this was all "normal," and nothing to worry about. At 6-months- old, my daughter began having trouble maintaining her latch. She would often slide off my areola during feedings, and she began to swallow a large amount of air. My nipples became sore again and there were teeth marks on my breast where she was holding on with her new top front teeth.

At 9 months, she baby was evaluated for a lip-tie, which was released. The ENT denied that there was a tongue-tie. When her daughter was 13-months-old, she was still gagging on food.

By 13 months of life, I had realized that two physicians and an IBCLC, and I had all missed her tongue-tie. I was able to find a dentist who was willing to evaluate her and release her posterior tongue-tie at 15 months, and we worked with an excellent Physical Therapist, who performed manual therapy to release myofascial restrictions, and showed us exercise to habilitate her tongue movement. Five weeks after her release, she stopped gagging on food, and she was able to protect her airway. She nursed to 2 years of life, when I weaned her.

Jacqueline's youngest child also had a tongue-tie. Although her latch looked fine, she knew something was off because her nipple hurt, and the latch was "not quite right." Jacqueline had been an IBCLC for 2 years, and had spent the majority her time researching and assessing tongue-ties. A physical therapist diagnosed tongue- and lip-ties, and Jaqueline had to wait 4 weeks for an appointment.

> On the day her tongue- and lip-tie were released, I felt as though a mental and emotional fog had lifted from me. I was no longer in pain, and the improvement of her latch was immediate. My first born also had his tongue-tie released on this day, and he graduated from Speech Therapy 3 sessions later.

Jaqueline feels that the health care system minimized her concerns, and overlooked a serious problem.

> I do not think any dyad should ever have to suffer the way I did with my children, especially my first child. Mothers should never be told that nothing is wrong when they clearly know that something is. Regardless of who is providing the support, the mother's report is always right, and she should never have to endure painful breastfeeding without an answer and solution to the actual problem. As lactation professionals, we should not have to use a bag of tricks for continual temporary solutions.

Jennifer

Jennifer is a Registered Dietitian. Although a health care provider herself, her concerns were minimized. Her baby's feedings were going poorly, and the baby was readmitted to dehydration and jaundice at 8 days.

> I felt absolutely terrible. I was producing only drops. Thus, we began a rigorous schedule of breastfeeding, pumping, and supplementation. Even as she recovered, I cross-examined myself, wondering how this was happening, when I had a very successful history with nursing.

Her OB/Gyn and endocrinologist told her that they were not experts in breastfeeding. Her pediatrician said, "sometimes these things just happen. It wasn't meant to be. It's fine to quit nursing."

> When I asked about the tongue- and lip-ties my IBCLC had mentioned might be present, I was brushed off with a casual, "oh, they say that about everyone. She can stick her tongue out. It's simply not tied, and it's simply not affecting breastfeeding."

As someone trained in science, she was not willing to accept, "Sometimes these things happen" as a reason. She began a diligent search for answers. Two ENTs and one pediatric specialist all said, "no ties." She reached out to a physician in Canada, who had expertise in tongue-ties, and an IBCLC author. They helped sift through the nursing problems. After 7 months of feeding and supplementing, her daughter was diagnosed as failure to thrive. Yet, she was receiving sufficient calories. The pediatric dietician brought in a speech therapist, who confirmed a possible tongue-tie.

> I was justified in my concern! After months of being brushed off by the medical provider community, figuratively patted on the head, and sent on my way, I felt validated.

They chose speech therapy to address her feeding issues. It worked, and her daughter was discharged after 6 months.

> I returned to my pediatrician, results in hand. Again, I was informed that "ties are a fad."

Jennifer expressed her frustration with the health system that repeatedly ignored her concerns.

> This entire experience is testament to the brokenness of the medical system. Those who could identify my daughter's ties were essentially under a gag order. When I boldly went to my pediatrician, I was dismissed repeatedly. I nearly faced complete lactation failure due to my daughter's ties, despite good breastfeeding management and experience, not to mention my own research and self-referral to specialists. No wonder so many mothers struggle to breastfeed, give up, and blame themselves.

She appreciated that someone was willing to listen.

> Thanks for allowing moms like me to share our story, and for giving us a voice!!! This was such a hard time in my life, and very life-changing for me.

Kaylee

Kaylee was born in the 80s with a tongue-tie. No one tried to help her mother, and everyone told her to switch to formula. She suffered from a number of health problems that no one ever connected to her tongue-tie.

Her baby also had tongue- and lip-ties.

> ... but our IBCLC provider said there was no reason to revise since there was only minimal nursing pain. Her early infancy was very difficult, she would fall asleep on the breast, feasting on my strong letdown, and rarely emptying the breast. She had to be held all the time, but wouldn't tolerate being worn, rarely sleep more than 2 hour stretches at a time for the first 3 years of her life (nearly).

Kaylee kept reading and decided to have her own ties revised. She noticed an immediate difference. A few months later, she had her baby's ties revised.

> ... oh, what a difference in her latch! Immediately after the revision, her appetite for solid food increased dramatically, and she gained some much-needed weight. She was revised two months before her third birthday and my only regret was that she wasn't revised sooner.

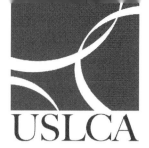

References

Agarwal, P., & Raina, V.K. (2003). Tongue-tie: An update. *Indian Pediatrics*, 40, 404-405.

Amir, L., James, J.P., & Donath, S.M. (2006). Reliability of the Hazelbaker Assessment Tool for Lingual Frenulum Function. *International Breastfeeding Journal, 1*:3.

Ballard, J.L., Auer, C.E., & Khoury, J.C. (2002). Ankyloglossia: Assessment, incidence, and effect of frenuloplasty on the breastfeeding dyad. *Pediatrics, 110*, e63.

Berens, P., Eglash, A., Malloy, M., & Steube, A.M. (2016). Persistent pain with breastfeeding: ABM Clinical Protocol #26. *Breastfeeding Medicine, 11*, 46-56.

Braithwaite, J. (2014). The medical miracles delusion. *The Royal Society of Medicine, 107*, 92-93.

Cinar, F., & Onat, N. (2005). Prevalence and consequences of a forgotten entity: Ankyloglossia. *Plastic and Reconstructive Surgery, 115*, 355-356.

Convissar, R. (2011). *Principles and Practice of Laser Dentistry*. St. Louis: Mosby Elsevier.

Convissar, R., Hazelbaker, A.K., Kaplan, M. & Vitruk, P. (2017). *Color Atlas of Infant Tongue-Tie and Lip-Tie Laser Frenectomy*. Columbus: PanSophia Press.

Coryllos, E., Watson Genna, C., & Salloum, A. (2004). Congenital tongue-tie and its impact on breastfeeding. Breastfeeding: Best for Mother and Baby, American Academy of Pediatrics, *Summer*, 1-6.

Coryllos, E.V., Watson Genna, C., LeVan Fram, J. (2013). Minimally invasive treatment for posterior tongue-tie (The Hidden Tongue-Tie). In C. Watson Genna (Ed.), *Supporting sucking skills* (pp. 243-251). Sudbury, MA: Jones and Bartlett Learning.

Douglas, P.S., & Hill, P.S. (2013). A neurobiological model for cry-fuss problems in the first three to four months of life. *Medical Hypotheses, 81*, 816-822.

Douglas, P.S., & Keogh, R. (2017, under review). Gestalt breastfeeding: Helping women optimise positional stability and intra-oral breast tissue volume for effective, pain-free milk transfer.

Fletcher, S.G., & Daly, D.A. (1974). Sublingual dimensions. *Archives of Otolaryngology, 99*, 292-296.

Fletcher, S.G., & Meldrum, J.R. (1968). Lingual function and relative length of the lingual frenum. *Journal of Speech and Hearing Research, 11*, 382-390.

Flinck, A., Paludan, A., Matsson, L., Holm, A.K., & Axelsson, I. (1994). Oral findings in a group of newborn Swedish children. *International Journal of Paediatrics, 4*(2), 67-73.

Forster, D., McLachlan, H., Lumley, J., Beanland, C., Waldenstrom, U., & Amir, L. (2004). Two mid-pregnancy interventions to increase the initiation and duration of breastfeeding: a randomized controlled trial. *Birth, 31*, 176-182.

Francis, D.O., Krishnaswami, S., & McPheeters, M. (2015). Treatment of ankyloglossia and breastfeeding outcomes: A systematic review. *Pediatrics, 135*(6), e1467-e1474.

Frymann, V. (1966). Relation of disturbances of craniosacral mechanisms to symptomatology of the newborn: Study of 1,250 infants. *JAOA, 66*, 1059-1075.

Gabbiani, G. (2003). The myofibroblast in wound healing and fibroconnective disease. *Journal of Pathology, 200*, 500-503.

Gabbiani, G. (2004). The evolution of the myofibroblast concept: a key cell for wound healing and fibrotic disease. *Giornale Di Gerontologia, 52*, 280-282.

Garcia Pola, J., Gonzalez Garcia, M., Garcia Martin, J.M., Gallas, M., & Leston, J.S. (2002). A study of pathology associated with short lingual frenum. *Journal of Dentistry for Children, 69*, 59-63.

Geddes, D.T., & Sakalidis, V.S. (2016). Ultrasound imaging of breastfeeding - a window to the inside: methodology, normal appearances, and application. *Journal of Human Lactation*, Doi:10.1177/0890334415626152.González Jiménez, D., Costa Romero, M., Riaño Galán, I., González Martínez, M., Rodríguez Pando, M., & Lobete Prieto, C. (2014). Prevalencia de anquiloglosia en recién nacidos en el Principado de Asturias. *An Pediatr (Barc), 81*, 115–119.

Genna CW (2016) *Supporting Sucking Skills in Breastfeeding Infants*, 3rd edition. Burlington, MA, Jones & Bartlett.

Kapoor, V. (2017). (Ed.) *Tied to tongue-ties. New clinical tools for early life care: the Possums conference.*

Kotlow L. (2015). Diagnosing and understanding the maxillary lip-tie (superior labial, the maxillary labial frenum) as it relates to breastfeeding. *Journal of Human Lactation, 29,* 458-464.

Kotlow, L.A. (1999). Ankyloglossia (tongue-tie): A diagnostic and treatment quandary. *Pediatric Dentistry, 30,* 259-262.

Kronborg, H., Maimburg, R.D., & Vaeth, M. (2012). Antenatal training to improve breast feeding: a randomised trial. *Midwifery, 28,* 784-790.

Kronborg, H., & Vaeth, M. (2009). How are effective breastfeeding technique and pacifier use related to breastfeeding problems and breastfeeding duration? *Birth, 36,* 34-42.

Labarere, J., Bellin, V., Fourny, M., Gagnaire, J-C., Francois, P., & Pons J-C. (2003). Assessment of a structured in-hospital educational intervention addressing breastfeeding: a prospective randomised open trial. *BJOB, 110,* 847-852.

Lalakea, M.L., & Messner, A.H (2003). Ankyloglossia: the adolescent and adult perspective. *Otolaryngology-Head and Neck Surgery, 128,* 746-752.

Li, B., & Wang, J. (2011). Fibroblasts and myofibroblasts in wound healing: force generation and measurement. *Journal of Tissue Viability, 20*(4), 108-120.

Lund, G.C., et al. (2011). Osteopathic manipulative treatment for the treatment of hospitalized premature infants with nipple feeding dysfunction. *JAOA, 111*(1), 44-48.

Madlon-Kay, D., Ricke, L., Baker, N., & DeFor, T.A. (2008). Case series of 148 tongue-tied newborn babies evaluated with the assessment tool for lingual function. *Midwifery, 24,* 353-357.

Marchesan, I.Q. (2004). Lingual frenulum: Classification and speech interference. *International Journal of Orofacial Myology, 30,* 31-38.

Maxwell, M.P.R., & Fraval, M.R. (1998). A pilot study: Osteopathic treatment of infants with a sucking dysfunction. *Journal of the American Academy of Osteopathy, 8*(2), 25-33.

Morgan, D.J., Brownless, S.B., Leppin, A.L., Kressin, N., Dhruva, S.S., Levin, L. et al. (2015). Setting a research agenda for medical overuse. *BMJ, 351,* h4534.

Mueller, D.T., & Callanan, V.P. (2007). Congenital malformations of the oral cavity. *Otolaryngology Clinics of North America, 40,* 141.

Naimer, S.A., Biton, A., Vardy, D., & Zvulunov, A. (2003). Office treatment of congenital ankyloglossia. *Medical Science Monitor, 9,* 432-435.

Todd, D. (2014). *Tongue ties: Divide and conquer? To divide and prevent an interruption in breastfeeding.* Australian Breastfeeding Association Seminars for Health Professionals.

Todd, D., & Hogan, M.J. (2015). Tongue tie in the newborn: early diagnosis and division prevents poor breastfeeding outcomes. *Breastfeeding Review, 23*(1), 11-16.

Tomasek, J.J. et al. (2002). Myofibroblasts and mechano-regulation of connective tissue remodeling. *Nature Review Molecular Cellular Biology, 3*(5), 349-363.

Vitruk, P. (2014). Oral soft tissue laser ablative & coagulation efficiencies spectra. *Implant Practice US*, November.

Vogel, A., & Venugopalan, V. (2003). Mechanisms of pulsed laser ablation of biological tissues. *Chemical Review, 103*(2), 577-644.

Wallace, L.M., Dunn, O.M., Alder, E.M., Inch, S., Hills, R.K., & Law, S.M. (2006). A randomised-controlled trial in England of a postnatal midwifery intervention on breast-feeding duration. *Midwifery, 22,* 262-273.

Wattis, L., Kam, R., & Douglas, P.S. (2017, in press). Three experienced lactation consultants reflect on the oral ties phenomenon. *Breastfeeding Review.*

Zeinoun, T. et al. (2001). Myofibroblasts in healing laser excision wounds. *Lasers in Surgery and Medicine, 28,* 74-79.

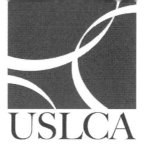

Appendix

Hazelbaker protocol

Function Item score: _____

Appearance Item score: _____

Assessment Tool for Lingual Frenulum Function (ATLFF)™

© Alison K. Hazelbaker, PhD, IBCLC, FILCA, 1993, 2009, 2012, 2016

Mothers Name: _____

Baby's name: _____ Baby's age: _____

Date of assessment: _____

FUNCTION ITEMS

Lateralization
2 Complete
1 Body of tongue but not tongue tip
0 None

Lift of tongue
2 Tip to mid-mouth
1 Only edges to mid mouth
0 Tip stays at alveolar ridge **OR** tip rises only to mid-mouth with jaw closure **AND/OR** mid-tongue dimples

Extension of tongue
2 Tip over lower lip
1 Tip over lower gum only
0 Neither of the above **OR** anterior or mid-tongue humps **AND/OR** dimples

Spread of anterior tongue
2 Complete
1 Moderate **OR** partial
0 Little **OR** none

Cupping of tongue
2 Entire edge with a firm cup
1 Side edges only **OR** moderate cup
0 Poor **OR** no cup

Peristalsis
2 Complete anterior to posterior
1 Partial **OR** originating posterior to tip
0 None **OR** Reverse peristalsis

Snap back
2 None
1 Periodic
0 Frequent **OR** with each suck

APPEARANCE ITEMS

Appearance of tongue when lifted
2 Round **OR** square
1 Slight cleft in tip apparent
0 Heart shaped

Length of lingual frenulum when tongue lifted
2 More than 1 cm **OR** absent frenulum
1 1 cm
0 Less than 1 cm

Attachment of lingual frenulum to inferior alveolus
2 Attached to floor of mouth
1 Attached between the floor of the mouth and the ridge
0 Attached to ridge

Elasticity of frenulum
2 Very elastic (excellent)
1 Moderately elastic
0 Little to no elasticity

Attachment of lingual frenulum to tongue
2 Between the tongue body-blade juncture and the tongue base
1 At the tongue body-blade juncture
0 In front of the body-blade juncture **OR** Notched tongue-tip

Scoring/Frenotomy Decision Rule

14 = Perfect Function score regardless of Appearance Item score. Surgical treatment not recommended.

11 = Acceptable Function score only if Appearance Item score is 10. Look for alternate cause of issues.

<11 = Function Score indicates function impaired. Frenotomy should be considered if management fails. Frenotomy necessary if Appearance Item score is < 8.

Martinelli screening

NEONATAL TONGUE SCREENING TEST
Lingual Frenulum Protocol with Scores for Infants
Martinelli, 2015

Name: _____

Birthdate: _____ / _____ / _____   Examination Date: _____ / _____ / _____

1. Lip posture at rest

( ) closed (0)   ( ) half-open (1)   ( ) open (1)

2. Tongue posture during crying

( ) midline (0)   ( ) elevated (0)   ( ) midline with lateral elevation (2)   ( ) apex of the tongue down with tongue lateral elevation (2)

3. Shape of the tongue apex when elevated during crying or elevation maneuver

( ) round (0)   ( ) V-shaped (2)   ( ) heart-shaped (3)

4. Lingual Frenulum

( ) visible   ( ) not visible   ( ) visible with maneuver*

*Maneuver: elevate and push back the tongue. If the frenulum is not visible, re-assessment is required at 30 days of life.

4.1. Frenulum thickness

( ) thin (0)   ( ) thick (2)

4.2. Frenulum attachment to the tongue

( ) midline (0)   ( ) between midline and apex (2)   ( ) apex (3)

4.3. Frenulum attachment to the floor of the mouth

( ) visible from the sublingual caruncles (0)   ( ) visible from the inferior alveolar crest (1)

Score 0 to 4: normal ( )

Score 5 to 6: doubt ( ) Re-assessment required in _____ / _____ / _____

Score 7 or more: altered ( ) Release of lingual frenulum is indicated.

Martinelli protocol

HISTORY

Name: _____

Examination Date: ___/___/_____   Birth: ___/___/_____   Age: _____   Gender: M ( )   F ( )

Mother's name: _____

Father's name: _____

Address: _____

City: _____ State: _____ ZIP: _____

Phone: home ( )_____ office ( )_____ cell ( )_____

email: _____

Family history (any lingual frenulum alteration)

( ) no (0) ( ) yes (1) Who: _____ What: _____

Other health problems

( ) no ( ) yes   What: _____

Breastfeeding:

- Interval between feedings: ( ) 2hours or more (0)   ( ) 1hour or less (2)

- fatigue during feeding?   ( ) no (0)   ( ) yes (1)

- sucks a little and sleeps?   ( ) no (0)   ( ) yes (1)

- slips off nipple?   ( ) no (0)   ( ) yes (1)

- chews nipple?   ( ) no (0)   ( ) yes (2)

History total scores: Best result= 0   Worst result= 8

LINGUAL FRENULUM PROTOCOL FOR INFANTS
Martinelli, 2015

PART I – ANATOMO-FUNCTIONAL EVALUATION

1. Lip posture at rest

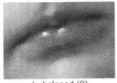 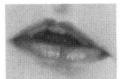 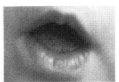

( ) closed (0) ( ) half-open (1) ( ) open (1)

2. Tongue posture during crying

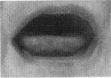 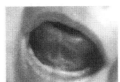

( ) midline (0) ( ) elevated (0)

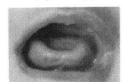 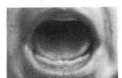

( ) midline with lateral elevation (2) ( ) apex of the tongue down with tongue lateral elevation (2)

3. Shape of the apex of the tongue when elevated during crying or during elevation maneuver

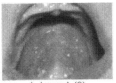 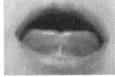 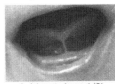

( ) round (0) ( ) V-shaped (2) ( ) heart-shaped (3)

LINGUAL FRENULUM PROTOCOL FOR INFANTS
Martinelli, 2015

4. Lingual Frenulum

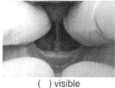 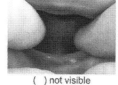 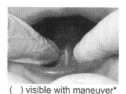

( ) visible   ( ) not visible   ( ) visible with maneuver*

*Maneuver: elevate and push back the tongue.
If the frenulum is not visible, go to PART II (Non-nutritive sucking and nutritive sucking evaluations)

4.1. Frenulum thickness

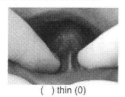 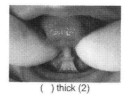

( ) thin (0)   ( ) thick (2)

4.2. Frenulum attachment to the tongue

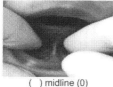 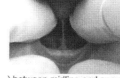 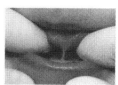

( ) midline (0)   ( ) between midline and apex (2)   ( ) apex (3)

4.3. Frenulum attachment to the floor of the mouth

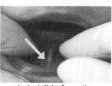 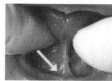

( ) visible from the   ( ) visible from the
sublingual caruncles (0)   inferior alveolar crest (1)

Anatomo-functional evaluation total score (items 1,2, 3 and 4): Best result=0 Worst result=12

When the score of items 1, 2, 3 and 4 of the anatomo-functional evaluation is equal or greater than 7, the interference of the frenulum with the movements of the tongue may be considered.
Release of lingual frenulum is indicated.

LINGUAL FRENULUM PROTOCOL FOR INFANTS
Martinelli, 2015

PART II – EVALUATION OF NON-NUTRITIVE SUCKING AND NUTRITIVE SUCKING

1. Non-nutritive sucking (little finger sucking wearing gloves)

1.1. Tongue movement

( ) adequate: coordinated movement   (0)

( ) inadequate: restricted tongue anteriorization, uncoordinated movements and

sucking delay   (1)

2. Nutritive sucking during breastfeeding

(when breastfeeding starts, observe infant sucking during five minutes)

2.1. Sucking Rhythm (observe groups of sucking and pauses)

( ) several suckings in a row followed by short pauses (0)

( ) a few suckings followed by long pauses   (1)

2.2. Coordination among sucking/ swallowing/ breathing

( ) adequate   (0)   (balance between feeding efficiency and sucking,

swallowing and breathing functions without stress)

( ) inadequate (1)   (cough, chocking, dyspnea, regurgitation, hiccup, swallowing noises)

2.3. Nipple chewing

( ) no (0)

( ) yes (1)

2.4. Clicking during sucking

( ) no   (0)

( ) yes   (1)

Non-nutritive sucking and nutritive sucking total score: Best result= 0   worst= 5

HISTORY AND CLINICAL EXAMINATION TOTAL SCORES: Best result= 0   Worst result= 25

Sum of the CLINICAL EXAMINATION scores (anatomo-functional evaluation and non-nutritive sucking and nutritive sucking):
Scores 0 - 8: there is no interference of lingual frenulum with tongue movements   ( )
Scores 9 or more: there is interference of the lingual frenulum with tongue movements.   ( )
Release of lingual frenulum is indicated.

Sum of HISTORY and CLINICAL EXAMINATION scores
Scores 0 -12: there is no interference of lingual frenulum with tongue movements   ( )
Scores 13 or more: there is interference of the lingual frenulum with tongue movements.   ( )
Release of lingual frenulum is indicated.

Contributors

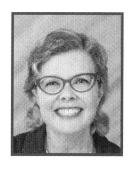

Kathleen Kendall-Tackett, PhD, IBCLC, FAPA. Dr. Kendall-Tackett is a health psychologist and International Board Certified Lactation Consultant, and the Owner and Editor-in-Chief of Praeclarus Press, a small press specializing in women's health. Dr. Kendall-Tackett is Editor-in-Chief of two peer-reviewed journals: *Clinical Lactation* and *Psychological Trauma*. She is Fellow of the American Psychological Association in Health and Trauma Psychology, Past President of the APA Division of Trauma Psychology, and a member of the Board for the Advancement of Psychology in the Public Interest. Dr. Kendall-Tackett specializes in women's-health research including breastfeeding, depression, trauma, and health psychology, and has won many awards for her work including the 2016 Outstanding Service to the Field of Trauma Psychology from the American Psychological Association's Division 56. Dr. Kendall-Tackett has authored more than 410 articles or chapters, and 35 books, Her most recent books include: *Depression in New Mothers, 3rd Edition* (2017, Routledge UK), *Women's Mental Health Across the Lifespan* (2017, Routledge US, with Lesia Ruglass), *Psychology of Trauma 101* (2015, Springer, with Lesia Ruglass) and *The Science of Mother-Infant Sleep* (2014, Praeclarus, with Wendy Middlemiss). Her websites are UppityScienceChick.com, BreastfeedingMadeSimple.com, KathleenKendall-Tackett.com, and PraeclarusPress.com.

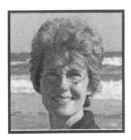

Marsha Walker, RN, IBCLC, RLC, is a registered nurse and IBCLC. She has been assisting breastfeeding families in hospital, clinic, and home settings since 1976. Marsha is the executive director of the National Alliance for Breastfeeding Advocacy: Research, Education, and Legal Branch (NABA REAL). As such, she advocates for breastfeeding at the state and federal levels. She served as a vice president of the International Lactation Consultant Association (ILCA) from 1990 to 1994 and in 1999 as president of ILCA. She is a previous board member of the United States Lactation Consultant Association, USLCA's representative to the USDA's Breastfeeding Promotion Consortium, and NABA REAL's representative to the United States Breastfeeding Committee. Marsha is an international speaker and an author of numerous publications, including ones on the hazards of infant formula use, Code issues in the United States, and *Breastfeeding Management for the Clinician: Using the Evidence.*

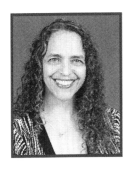

Catherine Watson Genna, BS, IBCLC, RLC, is an International Board Certified Lactation Consultant in private practice in New York City. Certified in 1992, Catherine is particularly interested in helping moms and babies breastfeed when they have medical challenges and is an active clinical mentor. She speaks to healthcare professionals around the world on assisting breastfeeding babies with anatomical, genetic or neurological problems. Her presentations and her writing are enriched by her clinical photographs and videos. Catherine collaborates with Columbia University and Tel Aviv University Departments of Biomedical Engineering on research projects investigating the biomechanics of the lactating nipple and various aspects of sucking and swallowing in breastfeeding infants, including objective analysis of tongue movement in tongue-tied infants. She is the author of *Selecting and Using Breastfeeding Tools: Improving Care and Outcomes* (Praeclarus Press, 2009) and *Supporting Sucking Skills in Breastfeeding Infants* (Jones and Bartlett Learning 2008,

2013, 2017) as well as professional journal articles and chapters in the Core Curriculum for Lactation Consultant Practice and Breastfeeding and Human Lactation. Catherine has served as Associate Editor of the United States Lactation Consultant Association's official journal *Clinical Lactation* since its inception.

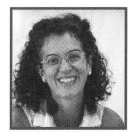

Carmela Baeza, MD, IBCLC, RLC, is a medical doctor and lactation consultant, specialized in family medicine and in sexual therapy in Madrid, Spain. She works in a private Family Wellness Clinic, *Raices*, in charge of the lactation program, and also teaches Natural Family Planning (Symptothermal Method and LAM). She is part of a workgroup on ankyloglossia, and is currently immersed in a clinical study to determine the effectiveness of frenotomy vs conservative treatment on posterior tongue-tie. She also part of a workgroup for the study of chronic breast pain and mastitis. She is the author of *Amar con los Brazos Abiertos* (To Love with Open Arms), a parenting book. It has two parts, the first to make the science behind breastfeeding easy for parents to grasp, and the second to address everyday parenting emotional issues that parents can turn from barriers into assets for their family growth.

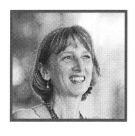

Pamela Douglas, MBBS, FRACGP, IBCLC, RLC, PhD, has been a general practitioner since 1987. She is founder and Medical Director of the Possums Clinic www.possumsonline.com, a non-profit organization and registered charity in Brisbane, Australia. She is also an Associate Professor (Adjunct) at the Centre for Health Practice Innovation at Griffith University, and Senior Lecturer at the Discipline of General Practice, The University of Queensland. She first qualified as a lactation consultant in 1994, and is author of *The discontented little baby book: all you need to know about feeds, sleep and crying* (UQP) www.pameladouglas.com.au

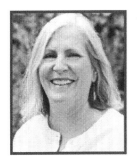

Alison Hazelbaker, PhD, IBCLC, RLC, has been in private practice for over 30 years. She specializes in the treatment of infant sucking problems using multiple modalities. In 1990, she authored the Assessment Tool for Lingual Frenulum Function. She also authored *Tongue-tie: Morphogenesis, Impact, Assessment and Treatment,* and co-authored *Color Atlas of Infant Tongue-tie and Lip Tie Frenectomy.* The second edition of her seminal book on tongue-tie will be available soon.

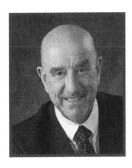

Martin A. Kaplan, D.M.D. maintains a full time pediatric dental practice in Stoughton, Massachusetts. He is a part-time adjunct clinical instructor in the pediatric post-graduate department at Tufts University School of Dental medicine in Boston. He has been an early adopter of laser dentistry, and has been standard certified by the Academy of Laser dentistry since 2003, and has earned Fellowship status. He has lectured nationally and internationally, and has co-authored several dental articles and been a contributing author in several dental texts. Dr. Kaplan was instrumental in developing the first in the country comprehensive Infant Laser Frenotomy class, which is co-presented with Dr. Alison Hazelbaker and Dr. Robert Convissar at Tufts University Dental/Medical Center in Boston. He recently completed his testing to become a Diplomate of the American Board of Laser Surgery and is currently the director of Dental Laser Surgery for the board.

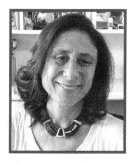

Irene Queiroz Marchesan, PhD, SLP, is a Research Associate at CEFAC, Department of Orofacial Myotherapy. She is a reference in Orofacial Myology. She has over 35 years of experience in research and clinical practice in Brazil. As a professor, she has visited several countries sharing her knowledge and experience. She has published books, book chapters, and papers on Orofacial Myology.

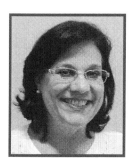

Roberta Lopes de Castro Martinelli, MS, SLP, has a clinical background in Speech-Language Pathology with a specialization in Orofacial Myotherapy. She works at the Department of child care in a Brazilian Public Hospital. Her main research area is Oromyofunctional disorders. She has published papers on her research field.

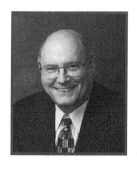

James G. Murphy, MD, FAAP, FABM, IBCLC, RLC, served 25 years on active duty as a physician with the US Navy, 12 years as a contract pediatrician with the US Navy and 6 years as a Government Service Medical Officer with the Navy in San Diego, CA, until retiring from government service on 9-30-13. He is a Fellow of the American Academy of Pediatrics, a Fellow of the Academy of Breastfeeding Medicine, Immediate Past President of the San Diego County Breastfeeding Coalition, a former Governing Council member of the International Affiliation of Tongue-Tie Professionals, a member of the International Lactation Consultants Association and, since 2009, an Internationally Board Certified Lactation Consultant. Dr Murphy began performing lingual frenulotomies in Oct 2003, and has performed over 4000 of these procedures to date including posterior sub-mucosal fibrous bands. He has also performed over 600 upper lip frenotomies using sterile scissors and laser. He is the owner of Breastfeeding Fixers, in Solana Beach, CA, which opened its doors on 14 April 2014, and is limited to releasing tongue and lip ties in infants, toddlers, adolescents, and adults.

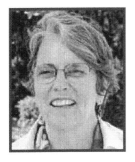 **Christina Smillie, MD, FAAP, IBCLC, RLC, FABM,** is an American pediatrician who founded in 1996 the first private medical practice in the USA devoted to the specialty of breastfeeding medicine. Board certified by both the American Board of Pediatrics in 1983, and by the International Board of Lactation Consultant Examiners in 1995, she values her continuing education from colleagues, research, and breastfeeding babies and their mothers. She's been a member of the Academy of Breastfeeding Medicine since 1996, and an ABM Fellow since 2002. She has served on La Leche League International's Health Advisory Council for over a decade. Dr. Smillie speaks nationally and internationally about the clinical management of a wide variety of breastfeeding issues, always stressing the role of the motherbaby as a single psychoneurobiological system, and emphasizing the innate instincts underlying both maternal and infant competence.

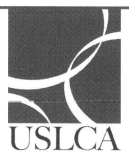

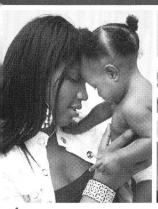
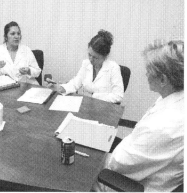
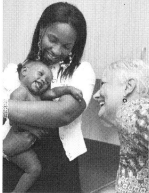

The U.S. Lactation Consultant Association Presents
Clinical Lactation Monographs

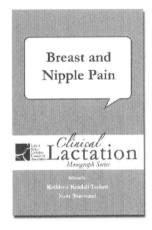
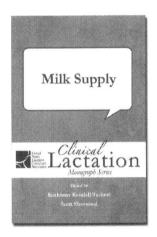
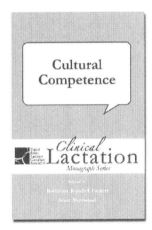
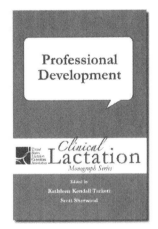

Praeclarus Press
Excellence in Women's Health

www.PraeclarusPress.com

Breastfeeding Titles from Praeclarus Press

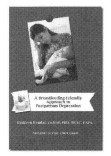
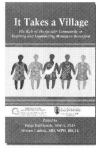
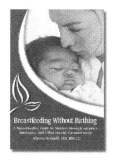

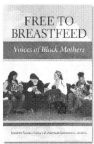
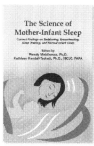
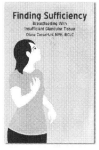

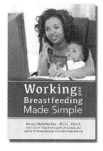
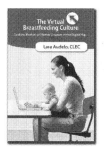

Praeclarus Press
Excellence in Women's Health

www.PraeclarusPress.com

Printed in Great Britain
by Amazon

78554840R00086